AS WE GROW TOGETHER FOR EXPECTANT COUPLES

AS WE GROW TOGETHER
FOR EXPECTANT COUPLES

BIBLE STUDY

HIS WORKBOOK

AS WE GROW TOGETHER FOR EXPECTANT COUPLES

AS WE GROW TOGETHER
FOR EXPECTANT COUPLES

BIBLE STUDY

HIS WORKBOOK

By

Minister Onedia N. Gage

As We Grow Together for Expectant Couples

OTHER BOOKS BY ONEDIA N. GAGE, PH. D.

Are You Ready for 9th Grade . . . Again? A Family's Guide to Success
As We Grow Together Daily Devotional for Expectant Couples
As We Grow Together Prayer Journal for Expectant Couples
As We Grow Together: Bible Study for Expectant Couples Her Workbook
The Best 40 Days of Your Life: A Journey of Spiritual Renewal
The Blue Print: Poetry for the Soul
From Two to One: The Notebook for the Christian Couple
Hannah' Voice: Powerful Lessons in Prayer
Her Story: The Legacy of Her Fight Daily Devotional
Her Story: The Legacy of Her Fight The Legacy Journal
Her Story: The Legacy of Her Fight Prayers and Journal
ILY! A Mother Daughter Relationship Workbook
In Her Own Words: Notebook for the Christian Woman
In Purple Ink: Poetry for the Spirit
The Intensive Retreat for Couples for Her
The Intensive Retreat for Couples for Him
Living a Whole Life: Sermons which Promote, Prompt and Provoke Life
Love Letters to God from a Teenage Girl
The Measure of a Woman: The Details of Her Soul
The Notebook: For Me, About Me, By Me
The Notebook for the Christian Teen
On This Journey Daily Devotional for Young People
On This Journey Prayer Journal for Young People
On This Journey Prayer Journal for Young People, Vol 2
One Day More Than We Deserve Prayer Journal for the Growing Christian
Promises, Promises: A Christian Novel
Tools for These Times: Timely Sermons for Uncertain Times
With An Anointed Voice: The Power of Prayer
Yielded and Submitted: A Woman's Journey for a Life Dedicated to God
Yielded and Submitted: A Woman's Journey for a Life Dedicated to God Intimate Study
Yielded and Submitted: A Woman's Journey for a Life Dedicated to God Prayers and Journal

LIBRARY OF CONGRESS

As We Grow Together:

The Bible Study for the Expectant Couples His Workbook

All Rights Reserved © 2016

Onedia N. Gage

No part of this of book may be reproduced or transmitted in
Any form or by any means, graphic, electronic, or mechanical,
Including photocopying, recording, taping, or by any
Information storage or retrieval system, without the
Permission in writing from the publisher.

Purple Ink, Inc. Press
For Information address:
Purple Ink, Inc
P O Box 300113
Houston, TX 77230

www.purpleink.net ♦ www.onediagage.com

onediagage@purpleink.net ♦ onediagage@onediagage.com

ISBN: 978-1-939119-19-3

Printed in United States

DEDICATION

To Hillary and Nehemiah

For teaching me these lessons

And sharing your childhood wisdom with me.

I love you and hopefully your wisdom will come in

Handy for my grandchildren and great-grandchildren

and all future generations.

AS WE GROW TOGETHER FOR EXPECTANT COUPLES

GOD'S WORDS

God blessed them and said to them, "Be fruitful and increase in number; fill the earth and subdue it."

Genesis 1:28a

You will be with child and give birth to a son, and you are to give Him the name Jesus.

Luke 1:31

Blessed is she who has believed that what the Lord has said to her will be accomplished.

Luke 1:45

AS WE GROW TOGETHER FOR EXPECTANT COUPLES

Dear God,

Lord God, I pray for these men daily, as fathers daily. As men, they need to hear from You. Lord, I thank You for hearing them. Lord, thank you for making them Dads. Lord, Your word says that You would fight my battles if I would just be still, so I know that You will help them to be a great Dad.

Lord, thank You for forgiving us of our sins and there are so many of them. I really love You but You may not know it because I am disobedient so often. I thank You for being God and God alone.

Lord, please teach me how to worship You better where my worship is pleasing to Your sight. I thank You right now Lord for loving me better than I could ever love myself.

Lord, thank You for holding me when I am happy, confused and at my wits end while parenting. Thank You for keeping me while I am in the valley and reminding me of Your presence and omnipotence when I am on the mountain. I am going to need Your hand of protection around me as I progress because I am certain to get myself in some trouble as I travel on this journey.

Lord, as I forgive others, help me to forgive myself. I need to forgive myself so that I can love and forgive others. Lord, teach me to love better and more completely and more authentically. Lord, I really want to be the best woman that You have made me. I need You, God!

Lord, thank You for time to study, the craving for me to seek Your face and Your heart and the ability to pray to You. Lord, help me to pray to You with all of my heart. Thank You for allowing me to come to You with all that I am and all that I am not. I need Your help with opening my heart to Your Words, Your message, Your messenger and all that You have in store for me.

I pray for these blessings in Jesus' name.

Amen.

AS WE GROW TOGETHER FOR EXPECTANT COUPLES

His Workbook

Dear Dad,

Thank you for selecting **As We Grow Together** as your workbook study during your pregnancy. You are truly embarking on a blessing. Your pregnancy is a beautifully blessed time in your life. This special time in your life also needs to be a time of prayer, study, mediation, forgiveness and reflection.

The time passes more quickly than you realize. Pregnancy is also God's tool which He uses to teach us that nothing is forever and great things come to those who wait on the Lord. Pregnancy is also His message that He can do great things through us when we are submissive and obedient. And let His will be done in our lives. He has it all planned and timed out. He just needs our participation.

God sent His instruction to write this concept through a great friend. She called me on a Sunday to tell me she was pregnant. At the same time, I was pregnant and another great friend was pregnant, also. She told me that I should write this after I reminded her of On This Journey: A Daily Devotional for Young People. What she didn't know was that He had shown me the vision. She was the confirmation I needed to proceed.

In this workbook, you will investigate who you think you are and discover who will be as a new parent. For those of you thinking: "but I am not a new parent," I beg to differ. You are a new parent each time you parent. In between children, we grow, change, learn and decide to be different parents. So you will parent differently. Lastly, you are new to that little one and that little one is new to you. While experience is the best teacher, most of our experiences demand our change.

Enjoy this time. Use it wisely. Nothing can get time back. Enjoy all the intimate moments you can with your mate because you will not enjoy that type of time together again ever. Your child will change and impact the way you spend time together with your mate and others.

May these words bless your pregnancy and the relationship between the two of you. In this devotional, I will often suggest you two are married, because you are. For the duration of the life of the child, you will intersect and be reminded of one another. So if you are not married and don't intend to be, proceed with caution. By the end, you may want to be married, maybe not to him or her, but to someone.

God Bless,

Onedia N. Gage

As We Grow Together for Expectant Couples

HOW TO USE THIS JOURNAL

Dear Reader:

Just a few suggestions:

- Mark your Bible with the scriptures that we study in the devotional. You may need them later in your life.

- Feel free to go as you need based on topics.

- Read the devotional daily. It is helpful for the two of you to both read the devotional. This will serve as discussion topics for you.

- Pray with your spouse/the other parent.

- Pray for your spouse/the other parent.

- Pray for your unborn child.

- Pray for yourself.

- Journal your pregnancy. There is a companion prayer journal to this devotional.

- Enjoy your time together.

As We Grow Together for Expectant Couples

18 | MINISTER ONEDIA N. GAGE

TABLE OF CONTENTS

Dedication	9
Scriptures	11
Prayer	13
Letter to the Expectant Couple	15
The How To Guide	17
Week One: Your Role as Mother	23
Week Two: Your Role as Father	45
Week Three: Your Role as Parents	67
Week Four: Vision: A Game Plan with God's Leadership	87
Week Five: Parent As A Teacher	107
Week Six: Faith is Required for Parents	127
Week Seven: The Lessons Ahead	147
Week Eight: Life is Short — Do What Matters	167
Week Nine: What Kind of Parent Would Jesus Be?	189
Appendix	211
Index	245
Acknowledgements	247
About the Author	249

AS WE GROW TOGETHER
FOR EXPECTANT COUPLES

BIBLE STUDY

HIS WORKBOOK

As We Grow Together for Expectant Couples

Week One

Your Role as Mother

Motherhood is an awesome gift. Your life will never be the same and it is no longer your own. Motherhood is also a tremendous gift and responsibility. Nothing is quite so rewarding as motherhood – not even fatherhood can measure up.

I certainly desired a child, but I didn't know I was ready. When we conceived, I was scared because I didn't know if I could do a great job. I had no idea how to do a great job. I had a few good examples, but could I be a mother, ultimately the mother God expected me to be?

In the next seven days, I give my seven stars of motherhood. These are my observations on the foundations of a great motherhood – the tools I've used so far. By the way, most plans you make may not materialize. Don't fear, though, the baby will have clothes to wear home and your husband can go home for the car seat, and without the epidural you planned, the baby will still come and you will still be sane when it's over.

Your role is broad, yet vague; rewarding, yet difficult; inspiring, yet revealing; powerful and life-altering. I do know this in her first 18 months, I have learned more than all of my life. She teaches me something new daily and surprises me daily, as well.

Motherhood is a journey, rather than destination. My last points are (1) maintain your sense of humor; (2) call your mother or mother-figure daily, and (3) your only real job is to feed her. No matter what happens, Hillary eats, is warm, has clothes and shoes, and I hold her and hug her so that she feels my love in her language.

Sunday	Your Self-Portrait: What Do You See? Psalms 139:14
Monday	A Godly Woman Proverbs 31:28
Tuesday	In the Spirit Galatians 5:22-23
Wednesday	Wisdom at Work Proverbs 3:5-6; 31:26
Thursday	Teaching God's Word Matthew 28:20

As We Grow Together for Expectant Couples

Friday   Powerful Relationship Builders (so a man thinketh)
                   Exodus 20:12; Matthew 5:5; Ephesians 13:19-20

Saturday   The Reap/Sow Principle
                   2 Corinthians 9:6

Week One — Sunday

Your Self-Portrait: What do you see?

Psalms 139:14; Isaiah 55:8

[14]I praise you because I am fearfully and wonderfully made; [8]"For my thought are not your thoughts and my ways are not your ways," declares the Lord.

Psalms 139:14; Isaiah 55:8

Many women overcome low self-esteem and others live with a low opinion of themselves daily. There is great news I want to share with you and I want you to share with others: we are fearfully and wonderfully made. God created you and your beauty, inner and outer; He created you in His own image. He created you to serve Him.

We are fearfully and wonderfully made. Some days it's hard to realize or remember but each day, no matter how we feel we need keep this fact at the forefront of our minds.

The following is your to do list:

(1) Stop criticizing yourself.
(2) Stop putting yourself down.
(3) Don't let others refer to you negatively.
(4) Believe you can do it – <u>anything</u>.
(5) Know that loving yourself is the least you owe God for loving you first!
(6) Take time for yourself.
(7) Care for yourself – spend a little extra time on your appearance when you can especially when you don't feel like it.
(8) Remember God loves you no matter what!
(9) Remember, the harder it is for you to love yourself, then it's harder to let God love you.
(10) If you love you, then it's easy for Him to love you.

This is a great time to correct your self-image. Whatever it is, it can afford to improve. And you will love the change.

STUDY QUESTIONS:

1. Rate your self-esteem on a scale from 1 to 10. Explain your rating.

2. What do you attribute that number to? How can we improve that number?

3. How do you define self-esteem? Do you view self-esteem as important?

4. How does how you feel about yourself translate into how your child feels about herself/himself? How does how you feel about yourself translate into how your child feels about you?

5. What can you do to enhance your self-esteem?

_____
_____
_____
_____

6. How will you help your child to have a healthy self-esteem?

_____
_____
_____
_____

7. How do you counteract the other parent who is causing the child's self-esteem to be negative?

_____
_____
_____
_____

8. Which 3 of the 10 to-do's do you need to work on first?

_____
_____
_____
_____

9. How will you help your mate enhance her/his self-esteem?

_____
_____
_____
_____

10. Who can help you with your self-esteem?

_____
_____
_____
_____

Week One — Monday

A Godly Woman

Proverbs 31:28

²⁸Her children arise and call her blessed; her husband also, and he praises her.

Proverbs 31:28

A woman who fears the Lord is to be treasured. This is the woman all people are drawn to. This woman prays and praises and worships God with her whole heart. She resembles peace and she operates with thanksgiving.

A Godly woman, who can find? I think being a Godly woman is a choice. We choose so many things. We choose to answer His call to Godliness. Sometimes, we choose not to answer His call. That's when the trouble starts.

At any rate, as women we need to choose to be obedient to God's calling. When we exercise in obedience, we exhibit our fear of God. Then we are called blessed. Then He praises us – his wife.

The short list of choices we make to be Godly:

1. Take real quality time and study God's word.
2. Meditate regularly.
3. Pray faithfully.
4. Love your child/children.
5. Concentrate on your womanhood – what God has assigned to you.
6. Plan for your family.
7. Seek wise counsel. Titus 2.
8. Remain faithful no matter what happens.
9. Remain gracious.
10. Stay your course.

Nothing warms my heart more than when my daughter smiles at me. She delights in seeing me when I pick her up from school or when I come home. I delight in her, too. Her smile blesses me. It lifts my spirit and encourages me to continue being the mother and improving my motherhood.

STUDY QUESTIONS:

1. How will you teach praise?
   _____
   _____
   _____
   _____

2. How will you teach respect?
   _____
   _____
   _____
   _____

3. How will you teach obedience and its importance?
   _____
   _____
   _____
   _____

4. Which 3 of the 10 choices do you need help making?
   _____
   _____
   _____
   _____

5. How do you define a Godly woman?
   _____

6. How do you define a Godly man?

Week One — Tuesday

In The Spirit

Galatians 5:22-23 (KJV)

[22]But the fruit of the Spirit is love, joy, peace, long suffering gentleness, goodness, faith, [23]meekness, temperance; against such things there is no law.

Galatians 5:22-23 (KJV)

When I read these scriptures for the first time I said ah-ha. These scriptures are important because these attributes are important to God.

Fruit is grown on a tree. This fruit is matured, or grown, by the Spirit. This fruit is born of the Spirit. The Holy Spirit is the spirit the scripture references.

For most of us, only one or two of these attributes are harder to achieve than the rest. For some, we may be having problems in all areas. We recommend that you work on one attribute at a time until you have them functioning well in your life. Functioning well in the fruits of the Spirit stimulates the growth and health of your child. When you are loving, kind and faithful, your child will be loving, kind and faithful as well. Further, children emulate and imitate our mannerisms. They inherit, if you will, our actions and attitudes.

Second to God being pleased with you, our behavior should match the attributes of the fruits because your children are watching. My mother was bundled up with excitement when I shared with her we were pregnant. She then said the apple doesn't fall from the tree. So when Hillary doesn't stop until she can do something and see it to completion like when she wants to screw the top on the sippy cup or tie her own shoes, I am reminded of my own persistence. Any of these actions make me laugh because she will be just like me.

This insures that I will love, so she will love. I will be joyous, so she will know joy. I will be peaceful and a peacemaker, so she will know peace. I will suffer long so she will know that long suffering is part of God's will. I will be gentle and exercise goodness so that she will be gentle and know goodness. I am faithful because I want her to be faithful. I wanted to be meek my whole life so that I can be her example of meekness. Temperance requires diligent prayer and my temperance has certainly expanded so that she will be calm in the face of adversity and her enemy. They are who they see.

Study Questions:

1. Of the nine elements, which three do you need to work on the most?

   _____
   _____
   _____
   _____

2. What do you do to please God?

   _____
   _____
   _____
   _____

3. What do you do when you are having trouble with one element? What is that element which is giving you trouble?

   _____
   _____
   _____
   _____

4. How will you teach/exhibit these elements?

   _____
   _____
   _____
   _____

As We Grow Together for Expectant Couples

5. Which one is the hardest to teach/exhibit? Which one is the easiest to teach/exhibit? List them in order from easy to difficult. Explain.

_____
_____
_____
_____

Week One — Wednesday

Wisdom At Work

Proverbs 3:5-6; 31:26

⁵Trust in the Lord with all your heart and lean not on your own understanding; ⁶In all your ways acknowledge Him and He will direct your path. ²⁶She speaks with wisdom, and faithful instruction is on her tongue.

Proverbs 3:5-6; 31:26

The three scriptures call us to action. As women and now motherhood, God designed us to freely lean on Him and trust Him. By creation, we pray more, are more emotional and are mostly more likely to deepen our dependency on God more quickly than our spouses. While this may not hold true in all situations, the real learning is I deepened my relationship with God as a result of Hillary's birth. I knew I needed God more than ever when He blessed me with the responsibility of Hillary. Verse five spoke to me loudly because this baby was a new realm for me. Motherhood requires knowledge and wisdom, neither of which I thought I possessed. If He commands us not to lean on our own understanding about average or daily events, then you should not be surprised that this new event would require to fully lean on Him for your understanding lacks comprehension.

When Hillary was four weeks old, I was still trying to get her to latch on to my breast. I was pumping the milk but it wasn't the same. I was home alone. I was tired because I hadn't been sleeping well, if at all. I cried in frustration, loudly. I then cried to God that He would hear my cry and offer me some portion of peace. These three scriptures combined led to a better day and a better understanding of my role as a mother.

His gift of peace offered me relaxation, increased milk supply and ended my frustration. We deserve to lean on Him – He invited us to release our "stuff" to Him and trust him for everything.

STUDY QUESTIONS:

1. What does it take to fully trust God?

_____
_____
_____

AS WE GROW TOGETHER FOR EXPECTANT COUPLES

_____

2. Why are you not completely trusting God? When will you start to trust God?

_____
_____
_____
_____

3. Do you seek God first or after you have exhausted all possibilities? Why?

_____
_____
_____
_____

4. Define wisdom. Are you wise by that definition? What does it take to gain wisdom?

_____
_____
_____
_____

5. How do you share wisdom? How do you teach wisdom?

_____
_____
_____
_____

Week One — Thursday

Teaching God's Word

Matthew 28:20

[20]"and teaching them to obey everything I have commanded you. And surely I am with you always, to the very end of the age."

Matthew 28:20

Your role as mother includes teacher. You are her first teacher. You are her sole source for certain information at least for a particular period of time. You teach her manners, mannerisms, attitudes, points of view and other things through everything you say and do. Even though you may not personally teach her everything, YOU ARE RESPONSIBLE for what she does and does not know. YOU ARE RESPONSIBLE!

You also are her mentor. She patterns her life after yours for the most part, but this requires that you are able and available for that mentoring process. You model the behavior and lifestyle you hope she will adopt and emulate.

Teaching God's word to your child might sound like a great responsibility, but the first step is reading to her while she is still in your womb. Reading Bible stories and scriptures starts you on a great path. This teaches the baby reading, the Word and a love for God's word. When we find something hard, usually it's something we don't do very well or understand. This is your opportunity and head start to study more and prepare to answer the questions your little one will pose.

As you prepare, gather some tools to help you teach. Preparation insures your success.

Teaching requires a lot but teaching is only a by-product of parenting. Love is the hardest concept to teach. They have to see, feel and live with love to fully learn to love.

STUDY QUESTIONS:

1. What will you teach your child about God first?

_____
_____

As We Grow Together for Expectant Couples

_____
_____

2. What are the verses you will teach first? List 5.

_____
_____
_____
_____

3. Why those verses?

_____
_____
_____
_____

4. What are your two favorite Bible stories?

_____
_____
_____
_____

5. How will you increase you study and reading such that you can influence your child?

_____
_____
_____
_____

Week One — Friday

Powerful Relationship Builders

Exodus 20:12; Matthew 5:5; Ephesians 3:19-20

[12]Honor your father and your mother, so that you may live long in the land the Lord your God is giving you. [5]Blessed are the meek for they shall inherit the earth. [19]and to know this love that surpasses knowledge – that you may be filled to the measure of all the fullness of God. [20]Now to Him who is able to do immeasurably more than all we ask or imagine, according to His power at work on us.

Exodus 20:12; Matthew 5:5; Ephesians 3:19-20

I define honor as love, obey and respect for your mother and father. To honor your parents should be a given. Keep in mind that all of your teachings and wisdom came from them in some fashion. Further and perhaps, more importantly, honor is given to them not only when they are great and deserve honor but when we don't think they deserve it, we owe it because God said so. Do unto your parents as you would have your children do unto you.

If I think I am a warrior, then I am a warrior. If I think I am more than a conqueror, then I am more than a conqueror. Whatever I think that I am, that is what I am. So what do you think for yourself and of yourself? Do you think and feel in the positive or the negative? What you have within you comes out when you are parenting.

Meekness needs to be cultivated. Meekness is a gift to others. I want to be meek, modest and mild, while my power and aggression live in meek love. Meekness combines humble love, a quiet spirit, and a genuine heart. Can you be meek? Do you want to be meek? What's the value of meekness?

As we conclude today of the powerful relationship builders, we will conclude with the power of God, the best relationship builder. In Ephesians 3:19-20, Paul describes God's love as love with such a full content that once He fills you with love, it will be beyond <u>your</u> measure. We often box up God's love by our own definition, but our box is only big enough to keep a hamster alive. However, His love does not live in a box of any size. Now, He further reminds us that He also does other awesome acts that we don't see or understand. We live under the impression that we can imagine the highest that is possible but He has power that is at work in us. He gave us an imagination and the ability to ask but He also does so much more. We build powerful relationships because we are powerful and so are our relationships.

As We Grow Together for Expectant Couples

Study Questions:

1. How do you define a powerful relationship?

___

2. How do you teach relationship building?

___

3. What elements are important in building relationships?

___

4. How do you honor your parents?

___

5. How do you define honor of parents?

_____
_____
_____
_____

6. How will you teach honor of you as a parent?

_____
_____
_____
_____

7. Share one situation when you did not honor your parents.

_____
_____
_____
_____

8. List people who are meek.

_____
_____
_____
_____

9. How do you teach meekness?

_____
_____
_____

As We Grow Together for Expectant Couples

10. What do you think about the measure and fullness of God? Are you full?

11. What do you think for yourself and of yourself?

12. Do you think and feel in the positive or the negative?

13. How do you increase the power that is at work within us?

Week One — Saturday

The Reap/Sow Principle

2 Corinthians 9:6

[6] Remember this: Whoever sows sparingly will also reap sparingly, and whoever sows generously will also reap generously.

2 Corinthians 9:6

As a mother, I have reflected and asked my mother many days how was I as a baby, a toddler. So Hillary is clearly a reflection of me, because you reap what you sow.

Fast forward or skip to the future. Truth: You reap what you sow. If you sow love in her life by hugs, kisses, time spent, gifts and encouraging words, then you will reap love in one or more of those same ways. When you teach hospitality and etiquette, then you reap hospitable and mannerable children.

Consider this fact as well, sow what you loved most about your life and your family. These lessons and values offer your child a similar family and value foundation. Further, sow in him what you lacked or what you missed. If you wanted more time with your parents, then you spend more quality time with your child. Since you wished that your parents were more active in your education, be active in your child's education.

If you sow in your daughter's life those things you desired, then you reap the benefits for your daughter as well as yourself.

A final note: try to avoid living your dreams through him in the material or social activity realms. We all strive to develop well-rounded children we are proud of. Just be cautious of the cost.

STUDY QUESTIONS:

1. List 5 details that will you sow into your child's life.

_____
_____
_____

2. Because of your childhood behavior, what do you expect to reap?

_____
_____
_____
_____

3. What are your goals for your child(ren)?

_____
_____
_____
_____

4. What dreams do you have for yourself that you have not achieved and regret and possibly cannot still achieve?

_____
_____
_____
_____

5. What one aspect do you regret about your childhood? Why? Was there a resolve?

_____
_____
_____

Week Two

Your Role as Father

Dad. Father. Daddy. Pop-Pa. Whatever your child calls you, you are responsible for their growth, for their love tanks; for their knowledge and their behavior. Girls love you. Boys reverence you. They grow to understand you as their role model and example for their lives and leadership.

Being a dad has changed since you were a child. Your role at home will be different from that of your dad. Your dad may have never done the laundry or changed a diaper, but you will probably do the laundry, change a diaper or whatever your family needs of you to support the family. You need to evaluate what your family needs and fill that need. These needs will be new for you to fill but valuable to your family.

Further, you need to ask your wife what her expectations are. Actively listening to her and taking notice of her expectations and needs will certainly insure the growth and success of your family. I shared with my husband that I needed his help. I defined help as prayer daily, studying daily and weekly, talking to me as I need, taking responsibility for taking Hillary to and from daycare, and several more items. Initially, his increased responsibilities seemed like a lot of work for him. With all that he was responsible for, he wondered what I was doing. So he asked. I shared with him what my duties are; he realized that he did less but his role was equally as important and it benefitted me and the family. Knowing that makes him understand the importance of his role and duties.

Fathers, your family needs your undivided attention. They also need your investment.

Dads, you are important to the total success. BE PRESENT.

Sunday	Your wisdom counts James 1:5; Proverbs 3:1-2, 7
Monday	Actions Speak Louder than Words Deuteronomy 9:18; 1 Corinthians 13:11; Ephesians 4:31; Proverbs 31:28
Tuesday	Actions Speak Louder than Words, Pt. 2 1 Samuel 13:14; 16:7; Psalm 51:10; Proverbs 27:19
Wednesday	Disciplinarian Proverbs 3:11-12; 13:24
Thursday	Provocation Ephesians 6:14; Colossians 3:21

AS WE GROW TOGETHER FOR EXPECTANT COUPLES

Friday   Patience (Anger)
                  Ephesians 4:2-3

Saturday   Love
                  Ephesians 5:1-2

Week Two — Sunday

Your Wisdom Counts

James 1:5; Proverbs 3:1-2, 7

⁵If any of you lacks wisdom, he should ask God, who gives generously to all without finding fault, and it will be given to him.

¹My son, do not forget my teaching, but keep my commands in your heart, ²for they will prolong your life for many years and bring you prosperity. ⁷Do not be wise in your own eyes, fear the Lord and shun evil.

James 1:5; Proverbs 3:1-2, 7

Your role as dad and husband requires your wisdom. As the head of our homes, you decide on our life, often with our input. But God holds you accountable for our provisions, well-being, and all things that concern us, the family. You, as father and husband, need to be wise. Do you have wisdom? Are you wise? Do you seek wise counsel? What is the wisdom test?

(1) Do you pray before you decide on anything?

(2) Do you seek your wife's prayers on your thoughts?

(3) Do you study God's word for answers and solutions to your needs?

(4) Do you seek wise counsel through the wise persons who surround you?

(5) Do you communicate with your spouse your findings?

(6) Do you move strategically or with anxiety?

(7) Do you study and research all means for completion of your needs and projects?

Being wise requires growth. You need to recognize that God is at work at all times. This fact requires that you understand this demands that your anxiety is misplaced and unwise. Wisdom is no respecter of age. Learning births wisdom. Be present and available to God for His direction and guidance.

Be wise.

As We Grow Together for Expectant Couples

Study Questions:

1. Do you have wisdom? Are you wise? What is the wisdom test?

_____
_____
_____
_____

2. Do you seek wise counsel? Who is your counsel?

_____
_____
_____
_____

3. Do you pray before you decide on anything?

_____
_____
_____
_____

4. Do you seek your wife's prayers on your thoughts?

_____
_____
_____
_____

5. Do you communicate with your spouse your findings of wise counsel? Of prayer?

6. Do you move strategically or with anxiety? Explain. Does your mate agree with your self-assessment? Explain.

7. Do you study and research all means for completion of your needs and projects?

As We Grow Together for Expectant Couples

Week Two — Monday

Actions Speak Louder Than Words

Deuteronomy 9:18; 1 Corinthians 13:11; Ephesians 4:31; Proverbs 31:28

[18]Then once again I fell prostrate before the Lord for forty days and forty nights; I ate no bread and drank no water because of all the sin you had committed, doing what was evil in the Lord's sight and so provoking him to anger. "When I was a child, I talked like a child, I thought like a child, I reasoned like a child. When I became a man, I put childish ways behind me.

[31]Get rid of all bitterness, rage and anger, brawling and slander, along with every form of malice.

[28]Her children arise and call her blessed; her husband also, and he praises her.

Deuteronomy 9:18; 1 Corinthians 13:11; Ephesians 4:31; Proverbs 31:28

Prayer

Our children need to see us pray and in prayer. When they witness our prayer time, then they learn to pray. I learned to pray in church, and I teach by praying in front of others. Further, my husband became more confident with prayer when he witnessed my fervent prayers. Allow God to work through your prayers. Your family will follow suit if you let God be your guide and father's prayers are particularly impactful and inspiring to the family and important for the family's growth and well-being. I learned fasting at church, as well. I experienced an entire life change the very first occasion I fasted. When you lead by example through fasting and prayer, you as the father set your family up for enormous blessings. Your family discovers who you are when you pray. Don't be ashamed.

Maturity

You are the adult, no longer the child. Behave as such. I grew up with friends whose parents are drunk when they come home or are awakened to drunk parents arriving home. Let the "failure" of your parents be your growth point. Acting mature encompasses mature decisions financially as well. Remember, your role as parent demands that your financial savvy take several steps up to meet the needs of your family. One more thought: I manage a retail store, so I hire quite a few people in this small town and its surrounding area. One day this customer was shopping in the store and she was behaving horribly. She threw some shoes down and demanded one of the associates pick them up for her. She was yelling at the cashwrap. Let's just say that it wasn't a great experience. Six months later, without knowing it, I hired her son. Even after his employment, she continued her behavior. Now he's ashamed.

Women

Your children will treat people, especially women the same as you do. Be kind and compassionate and sensitive to your wife and daughters. Observe and ask questions. Invest in their inner self. The information you gain will carry you far.

STUDY QUESTIONS:

1. Which one are you: Do as I say or Do as I do?
   _____
   _____
   _____
   _____

2. What will you do when your child challenges you on that?
   _____
   _____
   _____
   _____

3. What is your prayer life like?
   _____
   _____
   _____
   _____

4. How will teach your child to pray?
   _____
   _____

As We Grow Together for Expectant Couples

_____
_____

5. How do you measure maturity? How will you teach that maturity?
_____
_____
_____
_____

6. How will you teach the importance of womanhood? How will you teach the importance of manhood?
_____
_____
_____
_____

7. How will you will manage those moments when you have to choose between maturity or embarrassing you?
_____
_____
_____
_____

8. What will you do when your child embarrasses you?
_____
_____
_____

Week Two — Tuesday

Actions Speak Louder Than Words, Pt. 2

1 Samuel 13:14; 16:7; Psalm 51:10; Proverbs 27:19

[14] But now your kingdom will not endure; the Lord has sought out a man after his own heart and appointed him leader of his people, because you have not kept the Lord's command.

[7b] The Lord does not look at the things man looks at. Man looks at the outward appearance, but the Lord looks at the heart."

[10] Create in me a pure heart, O God, and renew a steadfast spirit within me.

[19] As water reflects a fact, so a man's heart reflects a man.

1 Samuel 13:14; 16:7; Psalm 51:10; Proverbs 27:19

These four scriptures are awesome. They address what really is important: Your heart. A father's heart is important for the livelihood of your family. Your heart is a reflection of your motives. You are the head of the home. God holds you responsible and accountable for the course you lead your family. Because of that whatever choices you make impact the generations of your children and your children's children. You have to make sound decisions and have great judgement. Further, your prayer life is critical to your family's success as well.

God listens to your heart. God monitors your heart. God is more than fair. He looks for the good within you as well as He judges the impure motives of your heart.

How do you keep a pure heart? How many times have we asked that question? Prayer keeps a pure heart. God also monitors your intentions. In this day, pure hearts may be hard to find a mentor to cultivate. However, pure hearts are required by God. A pure heart attracts God and compels Him to exert His utmost compassion on your family. This compassion is important for your family. The Bible recounts several stories of God's wrath on the family and land when a man is functioning with an impure heart. Take heed to those Biblical examples, so that you make decisions with the purest heart.

Above all, your family deserves a pure heart – yours.

STUDY QUESTIONS:

1. How do you maintain a pure heart? What do you do to get to a pure heart?

   _____
   _____
   _____
   _____

2. What does your heart say about you? Do others agree?

   _____
   _____
   _____
   _____

3. How will you share your heart with your child?

   _____
   _____
   _____
   _____

4. What grade will God give your heart? How can you have a heart that pleases God?

   _____
   _____
   _____
   _____

5. Who has the heart that you respect the most? Why?

_____
_____
_____
_____

AS WE GROW TOGETHER FOR EXPECTANT COUPLES

Week Two — Wednesday

Disciplinarian

Proverbs 3:11-12; 13:24

[11]My son, do not despise the Lord's discipline and do not resent his rebuke, [12]because the Lord disciplines those he loves, as a father the son he delights in. [24]He who spares the rod hates his son, but he who loves him is careful to discipline him.

Proverbs 3:11-12; 13:24

God disciplines us because He loves us. You discipline your child because of love, not because of hatred, malice, jealousy or exhaustion. Discipline may be hard for you initially. Sometimes you may have a hard time deciding when to discipline or how to discipline. The important point is to discipline.

Discipline is not popular by any means. The grandparents are not your greatest supporters, but you have to remain firm. You have to decide to discipline your child and be firm in your decisions. Further, be firm with your relatives and friends about your disciplinarian decisions. You may need to discuss with your non-supporters how their lack of support affects you. Let them use this time to understand your motives and responsibilities as a parent. This may seem strange because sometimes they are your parents you have to talk to about this.

Lastly, God instructs you to discipline His gift. He blessed you with the child and He issued the instructions for appropriate discipline. He disciplines us with love and grace and mercy. We need to do our portion for the good of the life of your child. Further, when we are obedient, we are lifted spiritually.

Yes, it's hard to discipline, but it's harder for God – don't you think?

STUDY QUESTIONS:

1. How will you discipline your child(ren)?

_____

His Workbook

_____
_____
_____

2. How will you and the other parent agree on the discipline methods?

_____
_____
_____
_____

3. How does God discipline you?

_____
_____
_____
_____

4. What will cause your child to be disciplined?

_____
_____
_____
_____

5. How will you explain your discipline to your child?

_____
_____
_____
_____

Week Two — Thursday

Provocation

Ephesians 6:4; Colossians 3:21

[4]Fathers, do not exasperate your children; instead, bring them up in the training and instruction of the Lord.

[21]Fathers, do not embitter your children, or they will become discouraged.

Ephesians 6:4; Colossians 3:21

While this scripture states "fathers," let's apply this word to mothers as well. The world emotionally batters our children. At home they need, expect, hope for and should receive love. This love is represented through discipline, instruction, praise, encouragements and protection. As parents, we strive for the best of ourselves and our children. This can only be achieved with all the components working simultaneously.

As a parent, we have to decide to strike a balance with our children. Discipline does not have to resemble a drill sergeant, while praise does not mean overlooking their shortcomings or disobedience.

The training and instruction of the Lord includes asking them about their whereabouts, meeting and interacting with their friends, hugging, checking their homework and administering discipline as necessary.

One last thing, parents: decide to share with your child. Share your life with your child. Past, present and future. I don't know much about my mother's past and I wish I knew more. Keep your life focused such that your child is the main part, not the afterthought. Finally, prepare for her future thoughtfully and purposefully. I use one filter to decide to include something on my agenda: what are the provisions for Hillary? After that, I set limits on how many events/occasions where there are no provisions for Hillary.

Children thrive on praise. Most of us will have to add that to our daily routine, but you won't be disappointed that you did.

Study Questions:

1. How will you balance discipline and praise?

___

2. How will you instruct and train your child?

___

3. What are the 5 most important aspects that they need to learn?

___

4. Have you ever been provoked or exasperated by your parent? What will you do to avoid that temptation?

___

5. What will you share first about your childhood?

_____
_____
_____
_____

6. What does your praise look like?

_____
_____
_____
_____

7. How can you include your co-parent in the praise, which all of you deserve?

_____
_____
_____
_____

Week Two — Friday

Patience/Anger

Ephesians 4:2-3

²Be completely humble and gentle; be patient, bearing with one another in love. ³Make every effort to keep the unity of the Spirit through the bond of peace.

Ephesians 4:2-3

Children require patience. Yours and their own. Their nature is inquisition; they are also observers. They are imitators. They do what they see. They say what they hear. They are your reflection. The apple does not fall from the tree, but even if it rolled down the hill, it would still be an apple—your apple.

Your second charge is loving one another through difficulties. Bearing with one another requires constant communication with God. This includes disagreements and miscommunications. Bearing with one another means forgiving, praying for, loving and persevering with one another. It means weathering the storm with one another. It means parenting with one another. Just as a reminder, this also means that you will support each other's decisions.

Lastly, "make very effort" demands your full attention, demands your 110% especially when you don't feel like doing it. "Put your best foot forward" – an old cliché, yet applicable to this scripture. Our charge is to keep the unity of the Spirit. Our duty offers us the results through the bond of peace. What is peace to you and your family? Once you gather up your peaceful experience, then focus on the actions which lead to the results of peace. Nothing you have is worth more than God's gift of peace. God provides peace to those who seek peace and who strive to maintain peaceful lives. Further, God honors those who protect the peace which exists around them. When we protect the peace, we show God we understand and appreciate the value of His peace.

STUDY QUESTIONS:

1. Who is the more patient parent? Why?

As We Grow Together for Expectant Couples

_____
_____
_____

2. What will you change about yourself so that you can be proud of yourself and your 'apple'?

_____
_____
_____
_____

3. How will your child know that you love him/her?

_____
_____
_____
_____

4. How will your partner know that you love him/her?

_____
_____
_____
_____

5. Can you consistently bear with one another?

_____
_____
_____

6. How do you correct a decision gone bad with the other parent without embarrassing the other parent and causing the respect for the other parent to falter in the eyes of the child?

_____
_____
_____
_____

7. How will you create and maintain the bond of peace and the spirit of unity between all parties?

_____
_____
_____
_____

Week Two — Saturday

Love

Ephesians 5:1-2

¹Be imitators of God, therefore, as dearly loved children ²and live a life of love, just as Christ loved us and gave himself up for us as a fragrant offering and sacrifice to God.

Ephesians 5:1-2

When neither of you has had a full night's rest for the fifth night in a row and nothing has gone as planned, you still love your spouse. Also, you still love the baby, because at the end of each day, when she's asleep and you stare at her, you know that you will give all you have and commit all of your energy to her.

Living a life of love as a father defines sacrifice and defies all understanding. The lengths you will go and heights you will climb are immeasurable at this moment. Your life changes each day she grows. You demonstrate love through your actions. When you hug her, she learns to hug. When you tell her you love her, she learns to feel love. I could go on with these examples, but those two prove my point of the importance of your love's impact on the emotional health of your child.

Although society does not demand a loving man, God strongly demands a loving man. God set the ultimate example through Jesus and John 3:16. Could you be God? Could you be Jesus? Could God have trusted you like He trusted Abraham when He asked him to sacrifice his son? The answers are likely no to all the questions, so the next question is can He depend on you to love His gift like He does? The answer needs to be a resounding yes. Children are gifts – not inconveniences, not an interruption to your life or anything negative that discounts them as the gift they are.

Love the baby as the gift they are. God expects it and we want to discontinue disappointing Him.

Study Questions:

1. Are you loving consistently? How do you know? Do others agree?

2. How can you love better?

3. Could you be God? Explain.

4. Could you be Jesus? Explain.

As We Grow Together for Expectant Couples

5. Could God have trusted you like He trusted Abraham when He asked him to sacrifice his son?

___

6. What can God ask you for?

___

7. Does God think that you are a loving person?

___

Week Three

Your Role as Parents

Proverbs 4 discusses wisdom at length. God expects parents to gain wisdom and information through experience and reading. God also expects us to pray for wisdom.

God clearly explains our role and fully expects that we will carry out that role completely to His specifications. Parenthood is a gift and should not be treated as a burden. As parents, we are to offer God-given instruction to our children and lead by example. Use this time to clearly define your expectations of yourselves. Many times we have said, "I will never do . . ." or "I will always do . . ." Those statements, while at the time genuine, are poorly timed for first-time parents. First-time parents lack the necessary experience to anticipate the reality of the situations which will arise.

Use this time to unite intimately with God and one another. Let, allow, permit, surrender to God cover your anxiety, meet all your needs and cover your fears. God had a pre-developed plan; allow Him to show you His plan and use you to bring His well-developed plan to fruition.

Parents have very specific instructions from God. Parenting is not easy. We are stewards over the child and we are accountable to God for their lives. Parenthood is an awesome responsibility. Parenthood surpasses all other lifetime milestones. Parenthood should be cherished and for the gift that it is. Use this time to make a commitment to your God-given role.

Sunday	Parenting and Our Christian Lives
	Ephesians 4:17-32
Monday	Our Timing
	Ecclesiastes 3:1-8
Tuesday	Faithfulness
	Hebrews 11

As We Grow Together for Expectant Couples

Wednesday   Marriage – Honorable
                         Hebrews 13:4

Thursday   God's Blessed Assurance
                         Hebrews 13:5

Friday   Peaceful Parenting
                         1 Corinthians 7:15; 14:33

Saturday   Peaceful Parents
                         Philippians 4:7

Week Three — Sunday

Parenting and Our Christian Lives

Ephesians 4:17-32

[32] Be kind and compassionate to one another, forgiving each other, just as in Christ God forgave you.

Ephesians 4:32

Of the much and faithful instructions given by Paul, these qualify for parents especially. The cliché the apple doesn't fall from the tree is a true assumption for most of us. My mother is an only child, therefore not really able to share because she never had to. I grew up twelve years from the nearest sibling and so I wasn't forced to share either. So it stands to reason, that if I don't change some history, my daughter will not share either. So it goes with other aspects of life that our lifestyles will translate and impact our children's lives.

Verse 32, kindness, compassion and forgiveness are each critical for a child to reflect the same. These are traits we are expected to model if we expect our children to know these qualities.

Verses 22-24, you are new in Christ and you are new being. You are expected to act "new," by completely dismissing the "old." This "newness" involves each aspect of life – your friends, your attitude, your behavior, your decisions, how you treat your family, and on and on. Our Christian lives are important to ourselves and the future of our families.

In short, verse 32 is an example of love: Kindness, compassion and forgiveness are all attributes of love. They don't exist without love and conversely you don't love anyone to whom you are not kind, not compassionate and unforgiving. These are all characteristics that we need to offer each day to our spouses and family and children.

STUDY QUESTIONS:

1. Am I kind? How is that defined? Who agrees with your assessment of kind?

AS WE GROW TOGETHER FOR EXPECTANT COUPLES

2. Am I compassionate? How is that defined? Does anyone agree with you?

3. Are you holding grudges which you have not forgiven others for? When do you think that you can forgive those grudges?

4. How will you forgive your child when she hurts you?

Week Three — Monday

Our Timing

Ecclesiastes 3:1-8

¹There is a time for everything, and a season for every activity under heaven.

Ecclesiastes 3:1

As I shared, I started this during our first pregnancy. When we started trying for the second pregnancy, we didn't conceive as quickly as we thought we would. Question: Why? Answer: God's timing. There are a million reasons why God's timing is correct and my timing is simply a preference.

When you study, please read the rest of the verses. They reinforce the ultimate impact of God's timing. When we surrender ourselves to God's timing that is best for us. We are able to release all our anxiety because the person who truly has our best interest in mind is God. He knows completely what our future holds and exactly how we will handle that. While that's great news for us, it also means work for us, as well. Preparation is required for us to have great responses. Intuition doesn't come to an unprepared mind. Reading, praying and studying prepares us for the expected <u>and</u> the unexpected.

We usually fear the unexpected. But the unexpected is why God is the expert. He determined our level of tolerance and ability to stretch long before our births. He does the same for our unborn children. He knows when the best time for the baby to arrive is – the doctor and the calendar are just guessing. So expect with great anticipation, yet no anxiety because He is in charge and has it all under control despite our plans or efforts to assist Him.

When we function in His timing, we live wisely.

STUDY QUESTIONS:

1. What timing do you want God to change? Why? What benefit does the change have?

As We Grow Together for Expectant Couples

_____
_____
_____
_____

2. What would the negative outcome(s) be?

_____
_____
_____
_____

3. When have you been glad that God did not grant your request? Recount two situations.

_____
_____
_____
_____

Week Three — Tuesday

Faithfulness is Crucial
Hebrews 11

¹Now faith is being sure of what we hope for and certain of what we do not see.

Hebrews 11:1

Faith is a prerequisite for parenting. If you don't believe that fact, ask your parents. Verse one is evidence of each of our lives. Let me explain: thirty years ago, ultrasound didn't exist. Now that it does exist, we can check the health, gender, position, and other factors of the baby(ies). Thirty years ago, parents had to believe that the baby was going to be healthy but any health issues visible to an ultrasound now were left to faith then. As parents, we did the requested ultrasounds; however, we don't choose to know the gender.

That example seems simple, yet it relates to everything else as well. When we are growing up, our parents have to have faith that we are going to grow up the way they prayed we would. They had faith that we would. They were sure of the results they hoped for and certain that what they do not see would come into fruition.

Faithfulness is crucial to parenting. Successful parenting requires faith. Everyday. All of the time. In your most glorious day and in your darkest hour. As parents we inspire our children through our own attitude about ourselves, them and life in general. In order to inspire your child, faith is required. You have to believe the information you share and the image you portray.

Often faith could be hard but not impossible. In all of our lives we may think that faith is defined differently, however they are all the same. It doesn't matter the socioeconomic backgrounds or ethnic backgrounds or anything else. What does matter is that we each believe that we love our child more than the next parents. What matters more is that we want them to love God more than anything. Faith is required to want them to love God more than anything. Everything else we want from them is certainly secondary.

STUDY QUESTIONS:

1. How do you define faith?
   _____
   _____
   _____
   _____

2. What happens when your faith is at a level which pleases God?
   _____
   _____
   _____
   _____

3. What happens when your faith is non-existent?
   _____
   _____
   _____
   _____

4. How will you show your child to be faithful?
   _____
   _____
   _____
   _____

5. Share a time when your faith pleased God.

HIS WORKBOOK

_____
_____
_____
_____

Week Three — Wednesday

Marriage – Honorable

Hebrews 13:4

[4]Marriage should be honored by all, and the marriage bed kept pure, for God will judge the adulterer and all the sexually immoral.

Hebrews 13:4

What does our marriage have to do with the type of parents we'll be? Some people don't realize how your current lifestyle impacts your parenting lifestyle. As parents, you'll be required to change certain aspects of your life to meet the needs of your children.

This would be a great time to introduce some marriage "game rules" if you will. Rules such as we will never argue in front of the children, we will never include the children in our disputes, we will reallocate how we spend our time, can be instituted immediately and easily and with great reasoning. I have learned that what children see at home is what they learn to expect in the world. My husband and I decided that the values we wanted out daughter to know she would learn at home. We teach love and care at home, so she goes out into the world and loves people with hugs, kisses, greetings and other such gestures. She waves and speaks and hugs strangers. She doesn't ask for our approval. She may learn hurt and hate but she won't learn them at home.

Deciding and teaching are easy. Children crave our attention, love and time. You have been chosen to be parents, so God entrusts you to do that with honor. This honor starts with the two of you. God guides the rest.

STUDY QUESTIONS:

1. Do you know how children feel when one parent betrays the other one?

_____

_____

2. Do you know how children respond to divorce? What do you know? Were you affected by your parents' divorce? If not, who will you talk to that you understand the effects of divorce on a child?

___

3. What do you plan to do help repair a relationship if there is damage?

___

4. Do you understand that your relationship effects your child? Do you know that children sense and realize tension in the relationship? What will you do to restore peace and love and unity?

___

Week Three — Thursday

God's Blessed Assurance

Hebrews 13:5

⁵Keep your lives free from the love of money and be content with what you have, because God has said, "Never will I leave you; never will I forsake you."

Hebrew 13:5

When we decide that we will submit to God's timing and get ready for the first child, we really don't know how much they can cost. And does it really matter? When it's time for the second and all subsequent, we have a much better idea of all the costs, that is.

There also comes a time when we decide to stop having children because we can't afford them. Daycare costs are huge. I do agree. Other items cost, too. But we say to God is that 'Your gift is not great enough for You to provide what we need and for You to overcome those obstacles.' I struggle daily (maybe not that often) with is two children my decision or God's decision. I feel that common sense should set in and I should stop when I have exhausted my budget and I have implemented all possible sacrifices.

Arguments erupt on this topic regularly in marriages. The solution is prayer and trust, rather than logic, reason, common sense and selfishness.

On a final note, God has an override button. Don't laugh—it's true. Have you ever seen your plans turned around and usually the completely opposite of what you originally planned? How about couples on birth control who have children? What about couples who want children, are not on birth control and have never been pregnant? God has an override button. What He designs and plans, not one of us can change.

STUDY QUESTIONS:

1. How do you submit to God? How does God know that you are submitted to Him?
   _____
   _____
   _____
   _____

2. How does God know that you are focused on Him?
   _____
   _____
   _____
   _____

3. How does God know that you are committed to His will?
   _____
   _____
   _____
   _____

4. How do you handle the curves that God places before you?
   _____
   _____
   _____
   _____

Week Three — Friday

Peaceful Parenting

1 Corinthians 7:15; 14:33

[15b]God has called us to live in peace. [33]For God is not a God of disorder but of peace.

1 Corinthians 7:15; 14:33

Peaceful parenting means we parent using only Biblical principles, we stand firm in God's plans, and we remain parents, rather than friends. Referencing several scriptures, we find that we are not to provoke our children, we are to give them wise instruction and we are to avoid ungodly influences over our lives. We <u>must</u> study the word so that we can do these things. We <u>must</u> pray to stand firm on our decisions based on God's plans.

Peace comes and exists when we know for certain that we have done His work and at our best. Maybe this seems vague, however, the truth is He chose you as a parent – you didn't make this decision for yourself. Because He chose you, He equipped you. Sometimes it's hard to believe or understand, but it's certainly true.

Peaceful parenting means explaining, talking and listening until she hears you. You are on watch for the fruit God will produce from you and your child. We can't afford to miss the fruit or delay the fruit because we chose discord over peace. Yes, peace is your choice. Peace is His provision and your choice. The fact that He has the plan is reason enough to accept the peace. We don't have to create or execute the plan – that's the great news.

Peaceful parenting is available to each of us. Peace requires our participation and acceptance. Peaceful parenting influences peaceful children.

STUDY QUESTIONS:

1. How do you recognize God's peace?

_____

_____

2. What do you do to restore peace when it has been disrupted?

3. How do you self-correct when you are the disrupter of peace?

4. Do you think God will discipline you for being unpeaceful? Why or why not?

5. How will you demonstrate peace?

AS WE GROW TOGETHER FOR EXPECTANT COUPLES

Week Three — Saturday

Peaceful Parents

Philippians 4:7

⁷And the peace of God, which transcends all understanding, will guard your hearts and your minds in Christ Jesus.

Philippians 4:7

God's peace – above and beyond all that we can imagine or conceive or understand – is available. He offers us access, unlimited access, to His peace. Just like salvation, peace is free. Your children learn peace from you, as with other characteristics. Experiencing God's peace requires your focus on God and His will.

Being peaceful also means that we have a spirit of peace, rather than dissension and discord. Peaceful persons love harmony. They avoid conflict at all costs. Are you that person? If you are, your child will likely be the same. When I realized that our child is like holding up a mirror, I then turned up my best characteristics and avoided my worst. I want them to have the best of me. I want to be a delight to them, just like I want them to be a delight to me.

Yes, peace is your decision, a decision you make consciously and deliberately to experience, to be guided and live in His peace. Having peace, being peaceful and being drawn into peace is your decision. You decide actively to seek God for His peace. Peace doesn't just happen. You decide and receive His peace.

Your joy will be made new and complete when you receive His peace. Your joy will be full and overflowing when you live in His peace. Your children will live in your peace and they will be introduced to a lifestyle designed by God.

STUDY QUESTIONS:

1. How will you reach an agreement without disenssion and discord?

_____

HIS WORKBOOK

2. Share a scenario when God has provided His peace and you were wondering how peace is ever possible.

3. What happened that made you act intentionally unpeaceful?

4. When God provides His peace, do you share God's peace with others, especially the other parent and child?

As We Grow Together for Expectant Couples

Week Four

Vision

A Game Plan with God's Leadership

Status quo means not exceeding the limits or testing the boundary or going above and beyond to achieve the results. My vision for my family is everything but status quo. Your vision for your family should include strategic plans for fulfilling the purposes God has for us as well as meeting the demands that children bring. This is a great time to investigate your plans for the major benchmarks of her life.

The vision needs to fulfill a purpose. Some events relating to completing the vision will be temporary. A visionary acts without short-sightedness, but rather the long-term effects on some great, yet sacrificial, decisions.

A friend had her son six months after I had Hillary. She took a courageous step in her career and proposed and was approved to work at home. It was important to her that her son be home with her. She made the necessary arrangements for his care when she had away meetings and conferences but most of her work week was with her child at her home. On the other hand I went back to work at my high-profile career, thinking it was important.

Two different decisions. Two families. Two women. I wasn't wrong to return to work but could've made a different decision. Or could I? Different results. What is your vision? What will you do during the different milestones in his life?

Your vision and the related actions starts the legacy you pass on to your children. Because of your choices, you can provide valuable influence to your children while they develop their vision.

The vision you and your spouse share serve critical for the life you now share with a little person. So how will you structure your vision?

What does God have for your vision?

As We Grow Together for Expectant Couples

Sunday   Let's Examine the Questions

Monday   Let's Examine the Costs

Tuesday   Personal Testimony – Hillary

Wednesday   Personal Testimony – Nehemiah

Thursday   As I Compared Notes

Friday   What is Your Vision
                      Habakkuk 2:2

Saturday   Making It Happen

Week Four — Sunday

Without Vision the People Will Perish

Let's Examine the Questions

After the bliss and excitement wanes and just before (or during) the morning sickness sets in, there are several questions you need to answer:

(1) What will you name the baby?

(2) Will you find out the gender during the ultrasound?

(3) Who will be the child's guardian parents?

(4) Will you return to work?

(5) If yes, who will care for your child while you are at work?

(6) How long will you stay home with the baby? Do you have enough time at work to take off the time you desire?

(7) Can you work from home? If not full-time, then some days of the week or some half-days?

(8) Can you and your family afford for you to stay home for 6 months? a year? eighteen months?

(9) What happens if you are scheduled off 12 weeks and you don't want to return to work?

(10) How will your life be different with this birth?

(11) When can you employ some help? Parents? Friends? Housekeeper?

(12) How will you raise your child?

(13) Are there any decisions you need to make before the baby arrives?

(14) How will you decorate the nursery? Will it be complete before the baby arrives?

(15) Will you breast feed? If not, which formula? Why?

(16) And other questions which may keep you up at night or wake you very early.

AS WE GROW TOGETHER FOR EXPECTANT COUPLES

Some of these questions are not critical or life-changing but for those which are, let's examine them. First, pray for wisdom, insight and sound decision-making.

What is your vision?

STUDY QUESTIONS:

1. What will you name the baby? Is the name résumé ready?
   _____

2. Will you find out the gender during the ultrasound?
   _____

3. Who will be the child's guardian parents?
   _____

4. Will you return to work?
   _____

5. If yes, who will care for your child while you are at work?
   _____

6. How long will you stay home with the baby? Do you have enough time at work to take off the time you desire?
   _____

7. Can you work from home? If not full-time, then some days of the week or some half-days?

8. Can you and your family afford for you to stay home for 6 months? A year? Eighteen months?

9. What happens if you are scheduled off 12 weeks and you don't want to return to work?

10. How will your life be different with this birth?

11. When can you employ some help? Parents? Friends? Housekeeper?

12. How will you raise your child?

13. Are there any decisions you need to make before the baby arrives?

14. How will you decorate the nursery? Will it be complete before the baby arrives?

15. Will you breast feed? If not, which formula? Why?

As We Grow Together for Expectant Couples

16. What is your vision?

Week Four — Monday

Let's Examine the Costs

There are costs associated with the life changing event. What are these costs? Starting with question four, "Will you return to work?" If you say no, can you adjust without that income? Can you replace that income within four to six months? Can you generate that income from home? Can you live without your benefits? Can your husband's benefits cover the family? Can you be completely out of debt before the baby arrives? Your 401k contributions will stop. Can you increase your husband's contributions to not lose the gains for the retirement plan? After the increased deductions, can you live on the one salary? Can you take an extended leave which secures your position for the length of time you want to stay at home in lieu of leaving completely?

So if you return to work, when will you return? Will you have enough paid and unpaid leave for the length you choose?

Who will keep the baby? Daycare? Home-sitter? Nanny? Have you started the interview process? Do you have the list of questions to ask?

Have you considered all of the options of your career to include those positions which would allow you to work from home?

Have you considered all of the best possible options for your family?

Let's count the costs. The most important costs is what you achieve holding your own baby as often as you can until she is no longer a baby. She won't let you hold her long.

You will never get these days back. Use them wisely.

As We Grow Together for Expectant Couples

STUDY QUESTIONS:

1. Will you return to work? If you say no, can you adjust without that income?
   _____

2. Can you replace that income within four to six months?
   _____

3. Can you generate that income from home?
   _____

4. Can you live without your benefits? Can your husband's benefits cover the family?
   _____

5. Can you be completely out of debt before the baby arrives?
   _____

6. Your 401k contributions will stop. Can you increase your husband's contributions to not lose the gains for the retirement plan?
   _____

7. After the increased deductions, can you live on the one salary?
   _____

8. Can you and your family afford for you to stay home for 6 months? A year? Eighteen months?
   _____

9. What happens if you are scheduled off 12 weeks and you don't want to return to work?
_____

10. How will your life be different with this birth?
_____

11. When can you employ some help? Parents? Friends? Housekeeper?
_____

12. How will you raise your child?
_____
_____
_____

13. Are there any decisions you need to make before the baby arrives?
_____
_____
_____

14. How will you decorate the nursery? Will it be complete before the baby arrives?
_____
_____

15. Will you breast feed? If not, which formula? Why?
_____
_____

16. What is your vision?
_____
_____
_____
_____
_____
_____

Week Four — Tuesday
Some Personal Testimony

When we conceived Hillary, I had recently accepted a promotion. I thought it was great. I was wrong. I stayed home for eight weeks. We were on the road as soon as I could drive. I recall her giving back her milk as I was trying to get my eyes examined. During those eight weeks, I was lonely and alone. All the arrangements and help I thought I had failed. I had little sleep. It was a notable disaster.

Have a plan with a paid backup. Ask your family and friends. Hope they come. Pay the cook, housekeeper and Doula. Now enough of the pitiful. I didn't investigate the other careers I could've easily transitioned to so that my motherhood could've been easier.

At any rate, I took my baby to a daycare, and being unable to leave because she wouldn't stop crying. I had to call in that day. I have changed her schools 5 times since then. She is now in a Christian school that is great for her and our family.

What did that change do to her? I don't know but we have communicated about each move. I have promised her little change for a few years where school is concerned.

I have learned that I thought my life could proceed as normal. I was wrong. I try to recover and recapture that time but of course I am unable.

The sacrifice of my baby's time was not worth the "job" I kept and gave the wrong priority to ended when the location closed just after I gave birth to my son.

Establish a vision suitable for your family. One you will be proud to share. I'm not completely ashamed because I know mothers have experienced worse but I certainly want to share my lack of wisdom and how it impacted my family.

Final note: My most upsetting moment was when she took her first steps, I was at work and I couldn't leave. She was walking. I was working. The results of poor choices.

As We Grow Together for Expectant Couples

STUDY QUESTIONS:

1. What is your family plan? Birth? After birth? Return to work? What will happen if you hate your choice?

___

2. What do you want to do?

___

3. Can you and your mate agree on your desires?

___

4. What does that require to accomplish?

___

Week Four — Wednesday

Personal Testimony, Part 2

Nehemiah gave me more trouble during the pregnancy than Hillary, but the outcome was different. I stayed home for 3 months with Nehemiah. When I started a new position, he went to a home sitter. Simultaneously, I started a new home-based business, and published two new books. Now the home sitter was okay, not exactly the blessing I counted on. So we changed to a school for three months, in between those arrangements he stayed with me. He could stay with me because my home-based business allows me the flexibility to change at that moment. Besides I had learned from Hillary the importance of choice.

Now in his short life he has been to four places and will be landing at his last place for a while when he is 18 months. I know that change is inevitable yet I try to keep it to a minimum but I will not let the "change" stop me from making a better decision for my child.

I am investigating returning to work full-time but only if I am able to put my children first. My children like to socialize so school is good for them. School is great for me because I am a room mom and am really involved in their activities. This is what I wanted as part of my vision.

He will attend school with Hillary when he is 18 months. The school didn't accept infants. I found the value of school versus daycare with Hillary. They will both stay there until first grade. At which point, I will investigate what is best for them, not for my budget. I can always make more money. I won't ever get to educate or love or play in this moment again. A little redemption for a mom.

STUDY QUESTIONS:

1. What did you wish that your parents could have done differently for you as a child?

_____

_____

As We Grow Together for Expectant Couples

_____
_____

2. Are you planning to do all that you were deprived of as a child?

_____
_____
_____
_____

3. Have you consulted the people who are closest to you to get their opinion of your choices or possibilities?

_____
_____
_____
_____

Week Four — Thursday

As I Compare Notes

At the top of every mother's list is the best for my kids at whatever cost. Then we stamp "SACRIFICE" on each subsequent item on the list.

I referred earlier to a friend who worked from home when she birthed her son. She already had a daughter who was older. Then on the exact day I had Nehemiah, she birthed her daughter. She did My impossible – she QUIT her job. She cited the reason of it was best for my family. It was never her initial vision but it's what is best for her family. Could you quit your job? Leave your career?

It is only temporary. When I wrapped my brain and attitude around that fact, not concept, but fact, I could really understand how to move forward and QUIT my job.

We compare notes regularly about how the changes are affecting everyone and it seems to be going well. We agree that we enjoy picking them before rush hour. We like being able to see our children between the six's, not at the six's. I would be stressed out to get the daycare center before too late. I don't want my baby to be last to go home. It gives me my pride to be able to be at her school for school parties and school dinners. I want it to be that way always.

Life is short. Our life is designed to be full and powerful and impacting. We have to live orderly. Activities we participate must align up to the mission statement and vision. Some of it's hard but it's not an option. When I have treated the vision or mission as an option, I have regretted it, immensely, not to mention what it cost me.

Final note: When you do what's best for your children, you find no regrets.

Live a focused and refined life.

AS WE GROW TOGETHER FOR EXPECTANT COUPLES

STUDY QUESTIONS:

1. What will you intentionally change because of the addition of your family?

___

2. What is the new family plan now that a baby is on the way?

___

3. Who do you compare notes with?

___

4. What are you learning about yourself which amazes you?

___

Week Four — Friday

The Family Vision and the Family Mission Statement

Habakkuk 2:2

²The Lord answered me, "Write the vision."

Habakkuk 2:2

Yes, write the vision so you can measure the situation against the vision. This leaves little to chance. There will be times when you will have to hold your spouse accountable and vice versa. There are times when my friends check my accountability. No, it is not easy but is necessary. Include in your vision, your total vision of their life; what type of care, will they school – public or private, when, where, how will you feed her, and all relevant factors. Revise as needed but keep that working document before you so you remain focused on the vision.

As for the mission statement, we used the Franklin Covey worksheets to develop our statement. It is difficult to take either document and remind your spouse that even his dream that he has had most of his life does not match the mission or vision statements. It's hard to tell your wife that this career doesn't support the mission or vision statements.

Both statements require prayer and time to write and adopt. Set a deadline and meet it. Develop the statements. They really make life easier when you are making decisions for your family.

Both statements and even the need for the statements will be challenged from time to time. Stand firm on your decisions and convictions. We are all challenged regularly. I listen respectfully, hear the facts and then share why we have chosen our course of action.

My mother and I always conflict about the children being in daycare than when I switch them to another place. I simply explain that this is better. After the third move, she just listened. She doesn't even question me anymore. It wasn't about being right for me but for the children. The first time though, she challenged my decision and even insisted that change may have been bad and my choice was poor. I had to stand with my decision. She later said she understood. In the future, I shared my concerns earlier than the move. She had a chance to process the situation, then provide her feedback. She felt better and so did I. My decision never changed but the process was smoother.

The grandparents prefer to know the vision, too.

STUDY QUESTIONS:

1. Your family's mission statement.

_____
_____
_____
_____

2. Your family's vision statement.

_____
_____
_____
_____

3. Your family's goals.

_____
_____
_____
_____

4. Your family's values.

_____
_____
_____
_____

5. Your family plans. By Year One.

___

6. Your family plans. By Year Three.

___

7. Your family plans. By Year Five.

___

8. Your family plans. By Year Ten.

___

Week Four — Saturday

Making It Happen

As I said earlier, these are the hardest working 18 years of your life. This is a short window which seems so long. You decide on the vision, then you have to develop an action plan.

October of every year, I start to plan next year. I keep great records of doctors' appointments and eye exams. This way I can pencil those in and keep up to date. We plan for about 2-3 weeks, including vacations, birthday celebrations, where to spend the holidays, even the budget for gifts and events. I suggest you do the same.

If this is your first or even your fifth, when you add another person's agenda to your calendar, you just multiplied your workload. You've got to remember more, you've got to do more, you need more, you've got to plan more. It is your smartest move. PLAN. PLAN. PLAN. Executing the plan is its own project. Explain the plan. Share the plan. After those two steps, execution becomes easier.

Now you are accountable for the results of making the vision happen. Your little one(s) is counting on you to deliver the vision.

Remember not to be completely afraid to make mistakes. As young people, they forgive easily if you say "sorry." They forget most of your mistakes, too. So with that said, please don't spend much time on those errors. Do spend time moving toward the vision with love.

Often you will be questioned so it is a good idea for you and your spouse to become more unified than ever. Rare, but possible, the questioner may be your spouse. Remind him/her gently of what the vision is, how the plan was established through the vision and remember to be focused on the end result for which you are striving.

Keep focusing on making it happen.

Keep your word to yourself and your children and your family.

STUDY QUESTIONS:

1. The Action Plan for your family.

   _____
   _____
   _____
   _____
   _____
   _____
   _____

2. How will measure the results?

   _____
   _____
   _____

3. How will you define success for your family?

   _____
   _____
   _____

Week Five

Parent As Teacher

"More is caught than taught" is a phrase that I have heard more lately as a new parent than ever. Being in the new parent club introduces you to personal growth through reflection. You are your child's first teacher and you will be her teacher all of your life. She does what she sees you do and repeats that action or words. He is a reflection of you.

Your child learns everything from you until she starts school and visits others. Be careful, this could be a compliment or a complaint.

Construct your lesson plans carefully. Decide on your parenting rules carefully. Remember once you establish your standards, take a stand for your rules and beliefs. Someone will challenge your rules.

Our rules:

(1) No secular music in front of the children.

(2) Certain words/phrases are not permitted (shut up).

(3) Can chew sugar-free gum.

(4) Proper grammar.

(5) No violent television/movies in front of children.

Remember that we live by these rules before them so we don't create a double standard. Otherwise, when you tell your child to do or not to do something, you may hear the words, "But you do it." You won't be able to prevent all instances but those things you feel strongly about, you discipline yourself accordingly. My daughter watches us so closely that I am so conscious of my behavior, the good and the not so good. They do what you do. They say what you say. Would you like to see your reflection when it is less than positive?

As We Grow Together for Expectant Couples

You are the teacher. You are the model. You are the example. You are the standard. Prepare for the best. Prepare to be outstanding. What is your lesson plan? What is your strategy? Who will assist you? When my children do something that I don't necessarily care for, I call my mother and apologize for doing that to her.

As a parent, I study and pray a lot. Also, I have personally taken some of the limits off of my life. I have enrolled in a master's program for business and will earn two other degrees, one of which is a doctorate. I will do it and expect my children to do the same.

Sunday	Salvation Romans 10:9-10; Ephesians 2:8-9
Monday	Spiritual Gifts Matthew 25:14-30
Tuesday	Love John 14:15
Wednesday	Faith Hebrews 11:6
Thursday	Tithing and Money Malachi 3:10 (8-9)
Friday	Worship and Praise John 4:24; Psalm 139:14
Saturday	Peace Philippians 4:7

Week Five — Sunday

Salvation

Romans 1:9-10; Ephesians 2:8-9

[9]That if you confess with your mouth, "Jesus is Lord," and believe in your heart that God raised him from the dead, you will be saved. [10]For it is with your heart that you believe and are justified, and it is with your mouth that you confess and are saved.

[8]For it is by grace you have been saved, through faith – and this not from yourselves, it is the gift of God – [9]not by works, so that no one can boast.

Romans 1:9-10; Ephesians 2:8-9

Are you saved? Do you remember your transformation experience? Do you remember your baptismal experience? Will you share your experience with your children? How will they know how to come into relationship with Christ? You are their first teacher on salvation. Teaching salvation is refreshing. Coupled with sharing Jesus with your child, your passion for Christ should be evident. The passion for God is what you are teaching, developing and sharing. Your passion for God is truly on display when you are sharing God and Christ with your child.

Your child's thirst for knowledge should spark a spiritual renewal for you.

Often seasoned Christians become complacent and removed from the best experiences with God. I believe God uses our children to ignite the best of our spiritual lives through our children.

He will also use our children to hold us accountable to Him. He did that to my mom. She became more active because He used me to propel her into action. God has used my children to remind me that He is right here for me, at times when I began to doubt.

Teaching salvation predominantly depends on your lifestyle. It is mostly what they see, hear and feel, rather than what you say directly to them.

Knowing scriptures will assist you in explaining how we enter that relationship. Romans 3:23 & 6:23 are the additional scriptures needed to support the salvation.

Caution: it is extremely difficult to explain that mommy and daddy sin and are wrong sometimes. Proceed with care.

STUDY QUESTIONS:

1. Are you saved? Share your transformation experience.

_____
_____
_____
_____

2. Do you remember your baptismal experience? Explain.

_____
_____
_____
_____

3. How will you share your experience with your children?

_____
_____
_____
_____

4. How will they know how to come into relationship with Christ?

_____
_____
_____
_____

Week Five — Monday

Spiritual Gifts

Matthew 25:14-30

[18]But the man who had received the one talent went off, dug a hole in the ground and hid his master's money.

Matthew 25:18

What are your gifts? Are you using them as prescribed by Christ? If not, why not? If so, you have chosen to pass on the life God endowed you with. Part of our responsibility as parents is to pass on a legacy of Christ, which includes teaching how to realize our gifts and using those gifts to increase God's Kingdom.

Will they use their gifts at school and work? Certainly.

Teaching them to use their gifts for the benefit of Christ is what counts. I love teaching lessons on spiritual gifts. I love the transformation in those I teach. Most people simply don't realize. Once they do know, I witness a transformation in their lives. They start to work in the church, they do a better job sharing Christ, and they focus on what Christ needs of them. Further, they are better accountable Christians. They are more involved in church and fellowship with other believers. They have the tendency to be more knowledgeable about Christ because the involvement has increased.

The first way to teach use of gifts is by example. Do you use your gifts? Have you explained your gifts to your children? Have they seen your gifts in action? Have you invited them to participate as you use your gifts?

The second way to teach the use of gifts is giving them opportunities to develop their gifts. When you consider what they do at home use that same activities for them to share with elderly persons or other children, at church, or at the hospital or shelters.

When we teach spiritual gifts and teach giving of themselves earlier, we raise responsible children at an earlier time.

Start a legacy of giving back to God what He has given to us to use for His kingdom.

As We Grow Together for Expectant Couples

STUDY QUESTIONS:

1. What are your gifts?

___

2. Are you using them as prescribed by Christ? If not, why not?

___

3. How will you explain your gifts to your children? How will you help them understand their gifts?

___

4. How will you help your children use their gifts?

___

Week Five — Tuesday

Love

John 14:15

¹⁵If you love me, you will obey what I command.

John 14:15

Gage theory: "If I love them, they will obey me." I suggest this because obedience with any other source is temporary. Fear and intimidation only last until they leave home. Love lasts and teaches more, builds confidence and self-esteem.

Teaching love is based on what they see, feel, know, hear and experience. Why are we teaching love? "Won't they just get it?" you may be thinking. Well no. Love is taught at home.

I learned how to love and how not to love at home. I consider my home life and sometimes, I made up love. As an adult, I still love differently than most people. I love too easily. I love completely or not at all. I still think that everyone should love me, regardless. Does it happen – no. We also need to teach the source of Love: God. God and Jesus are the true and only examples of love.

Love and trust will become synonymous, even though they shouldn't. I have to teach how not to be so trusting with people – even her "friends" at school. She defines them as friends, while I don't. We then engage in quite careful conversation about love, friendships and trust.

Love is the foundation of who we are. Love is like air and oxygen. Without love, similar to oxygen, the brain and body doesn't function properly, creating issues later in life.

Love is nurtured. Love is an action. Love is really a verb. Dr. Gary Chapman authors a series of books entitled <u>The Five Love Languages</u>, one of which addresses the love language of children. He addresses strategies to love your child in her language.

Love is critical. Teach through loving. Live love.

STUDY QUESTIONS:

1. Why do we teach love?

_____
_____
_____
_____

2. How will we teach love?

_____
_____
_____
_____

3. How will we demonstrate love in a mechanism were they can learn to love as well?

_____
_____
_____
_____

4. How will you show them how valuable love is?

_____
_____
_____
_____

Week Five — Wednesday

Faith

Hebrews 11:6

⁶And without faith it is impossible to please God, because anyone who comes to Him must believe that He exists and that He rewards those who earnestly seek Him.

Hebrews 11:6

How do we teach faith? This may not be fair but hold up a mirror and check your faith. Do you have faith or do you worry? Do you fret? Do you need consistent reassurance? Are you overly anxious? When you pray, do you really give <u>all</u> of your burdens to God? And leave them with Him permanently? While we may not be able to answer no to all the questions all the time, answer according to your usual behavior.

Your child is watching your behavior, listening to your words, listening to the tone of your voice and feeling your emotional vibes.

Teaching faith is modeling faith. Do you believe in His Power? Do you believe in His will? Do you "earnestly" seek Him? Do you trust Him and His word? That is your exhibit of faith.

Faith is the evidence of what is hoped for but yet unseen.

Modeling faith is work. Waiting on the Lord requires work, real work. Faith is not thinking that God will deliver a job to your door. Faith is applying for each position where you are interested and knowing that God will supply a job based on your efforts. Faith is not thinking that God will make you debt-free when you acquire more credit cards and keep them at the limit. Faith requires us to stop spending, diligently pay down the debt and cut up the cards. Faith is praying and fasting in belief that God keeps His word. Faith is our refuge in the Lord. He is our strength. Faith is our thank you. Faith is us believing that He is who He says He is. Faith is knowing that what God has for you is for you.

Faith is professing the positive over your life. Faith is believing God and doing what He said.

Faith is modeled behavior.

AS WE GROW TOGETHER FOR EXPECTANT COUPLES

STUDY QUESTIONS:

1. How do we teach faith?

   _____
   _____
   _____
   _____

2. Do you have faith or do you worry? Do you fret? Do you need consistent reassurance? Are you overly anxious? Explain.

   _____
   _____
   _____
   _____

3. When you pray, do you really give all of your burdens to God? And leave them with Him permanently?

   _____
   _____
   _____
   _____

4. Do you believe in His power? Do you believe in His will? Do you "earnestly" seek Him?

   _____
   _____
   _____

5. Do you trust Him and His word?

Week Five — Thursday

Tithing and Money

Malachi 3:8-10

[8]"Will a man rob God? Yet you rob me." "But you ask, 'How do we rob you?'" "In tithes and offerings. [9]You are under a curse – the whole nation of you – because you are robbing me. [10]Bring the whole tithe into the storehouse, that there may be food in my house. Test me in this," says the Lord Almighty, "and see if I will not throw open the floodgates of heaven and pour out so much blessing that you will not have room enough for it.

Malachi 3:8-10

There are unlimited testimonies about what God does when we are obedient. Tithing is hard for some people; there have been times when it has been hard for me. I know it is something I must do.

There are unlimited testimonies about people who don't believe in tithing. They also have a long list of other Biblical principles they don't believe in. It calls into question whether they are truly Christians.

Tithing is an act of trust and obedience. Sometimes it's hard and sometimes easy.

Teaching it requires transparency. Place three jars or boxes in your child's room. Label the first as "tithes." Label the second as "savings." Label the third as "the rest." Do this when they start receiving an allowance. They also need a dream notebook. In this dream notebook, they gather up ideas for "the rest." Use this exercise to teach dreaming as well.

The jars will hold them accountable. When it's time to go to church, they empty the jar and give it to church. They will be proud and they will be disciplined. They will need to be reminded.

Tithing is one of God's requirements.

STUDY QUESTIONS:

1. How do you feel about money?

___

2. How will you teach about money?

___

3. How will measure the success of that?

___

4. Is this on the mission, vision, goals, value and action plans?

___

AS WE GROW TOGETHER FOR EXPECTANT COUPLES

5. Can you be transparent with yourself, your mate and your child?

_____
_____
_____
_____

Week Five — Friday

Worship and Praise

John 4:24; Psalm 139:14

^{24}"God is spirit, and his worshippers must worship in spirit and in truth."

^{14}I praise you because I am fearfully and wonderfully made, your works are wonderful, I know that full well.

John 4:24; Psalm 139:14

Worship is personal, yet your children should know that you WORSHIP the Lord. Hillary, my older child, loves worship. She taught her brother about worship. Worship is your reverence to God. Your quiet time, prayer time and meditation time constitutes worship.

Praise is more fun and more expressive. I taught Hillary how to PRAISE. She sees me clap, hears me sing and asks me if I am crying when I praise the Lord. She taught Nehemiah. He watched her clap and sing and dance before the Lord. Nehemiah claps, sings and dances before the Lord now, too. Hillary has corrected his dancing, as well. Correcting his praise aside, Hillary knows how to praise God and does so daily. My greatest accomplishment is that my children praise the Lord because they love the Lord. They learned it from me.

I have a rule that we don't listen to random secular music. There are certain songs, mostly ones from movies that they can listen to as well as instrumental jazz. Music becomes a part of your soul. You must monitor their, as well as your own, musical intake. They learned to praise because they see me praise the Lord in my truck on the way to our destinations <u>daily</u>.

Worship is the meat on the plate. Praise is the everything else, including the beverage. This is the description of a balanced diet. We cannot leave one of them alone. For properly living, we need both.

The Lord knows that we love Him through obedience, worship and praise. We were created to praise and worship Him. Don't let the rocks cry out in your place.

STUDY QUESTIONS:

1. How do you worship the Lord?

2. How do you praise the Lord?

3. How will you demonstrate/teach praise and worship the Lord to your child?

Week Five — Saturday

Peace

Philippians 4:7

⁷And the peace of God, which transcends all understanding, will guard your hearts and minds in Chris Jesus.

Philippians 4:7

God's peace transcends all understanding. Teaching peace requires seeking His peace. Keep in mind, understanding His peace is not required, since it's nearly impossible. Do you seek God's peace? Do you expect God's peace? Do you need God's peace? Do you want God's peace? Do you ask God for His peace?

Teaching peace requires peaceful behavior. Peacefulness requires submission.

Now let's talk about what His peace will do: His peace guards your heart and mind in Christ Jesus. The definition of guard is to cover; prevent from hurt, harm and danger; to protect from all issues and persons.

God protects your heart and mind. God protects your heart and your mind with His peace. God's peace protects our heart and your mind. With all that we encounter and face and manage and seek and cope, HE protects our hearts with His amazing peace. For all that we see, hear, ignore, persevere and feel, HE protects our minds with His magnificent peace.

When I start to meditate on those very words and consider the events that were an attempt on my sanity and designed to hinder my ability to love, reason, function and think, I have to THANK Him for His peace.

When I consider the unkind words, thoughts, and intentions of others to me, I consider His peace, which I do not understand, bestowed on me unexpectedly, and His peace overwhelms and consumes me.

Be overwhelmed, consumed and functioning with His peace. That is how a parent teaches peace.

STUDY QUESTIONS:

1. Do you do anything which will sabotage the peace that God provides?

2. Do you recognize God's peace?

3. Do you accept God's peace? Always?

4. How will you teach your child to recognize the peace that God provides?

5. How will you teach how to not reject it and to not sabotage God's peace?

_____
_____
_____
_____

Week Six

Faith is Required for Parents

In the childbirth preparation class, we did an exercise where we closed our eyes and picked from some cards. On these cards were printed on either side: vaginal/cesarean, no complications/NICU, long labor/short labor, etc. In all of the scenarios, the facilitator explained what to anticipate. Some of the possibilities were horrible but not impossible.

The outcome requires faith.

Our daughter was born at 5 pounds and 7 ounces. The team tried to explain all of the negative possibilities, including feeding her with a tube, and bottle, putting her in NICU, and they were the picture of doom and gloom. I had no problems with the pregnancy, or the birth. She was simply "underweight." I placed that in quotes because while she may have been in an area on the weight chart where they were uncomfortable, God is in control. They threatened me with all kinds of consequences if she didn't gain weight. She needed two ounces. I prayed over her with my hands on her. God responds to our faith, or lack thereof. Hillary never lost an ounce, gained the two ounces, came home on time and never visited the NICU, tube or bottle feeding.

What do you trust God with?

What are you believing God for?

Our son was born cesarean style. Not what we wanted or expected but truly necessary. The event means nothing once God has shown up. No need for panic or alarm. God's will be done. Submit and surrender. Consider it all joy. Yes, it is easy for me to say.

God blesses those who believe.

Trust Him with all – it all belongs to Him anyway. Give it all to Him – He knows it all anyway.

Believe that He will handle it all – He is in charge because it is His plans and design.

As We Grow Together for Expectant Couples

Sunday			The Faith Quiz: Can you Pass?
			Hebrews 11:1, 3

Monday			Faith: A Commitment to God
			Hebrews 11:6

Tuesday			Faith: Walk the Walk, Stop Talking
			Matthew 14:28-31; Luke 8:43-48

Wednesday		Faith: Sometimes Alone
			Genesis 12-Genesis 22

Thursday		Faith: Pass It On
			2 Timothy 1:5-6; Romans 1:12

Friday			Faith: An Action, Not Discussion
			James 2:26; Matthew 17:20

Saturday		Faith: The Final Word
			Hebrews 12:2; Matthew 25:21

Week Six — Sunday

The Faith Quiz: Can You Pass?

Hebrews 11:1, 3

[1]Now faith is being sure of what we hope for and certain of what we do not see. [3]By faith we understand that the universe was formed at God's command, so that what is seen was not made out of what was visible.

Hebrews 11:1, 3

Are you faithful?

Do you worry?

Do you submit to faith?

Do you speak as if greatness is possible?

Do you share the great things that happen?

Do you believe God will do what you ask?

Do you ask believing that God will answer and provide?

Do you pray? Regularly?

Do you fast? Regularly?

Do you have a prayer partner?

Do others know that you are faithful?

Do you speak with belief?

Do you think faith is important?

Do you know that God expects you to have faith?

How do you measure faith?

How does your measurement compare to God's?

Do your children know that you have faith?

Do you encourage others to have faith?

Do you know any scriptures about faith?

Do you move with faith?

When you consider your answers to these questions, would you pass if this were a test? More importantly, how does God grade your faith? Are you an example of faith?

In this week's introduction, I asked you two questions: (1) What do you trust God with?, and, (2) What are you believing God for? I want you to ponder these questions because you need to know and share the answers. I trust God with my "stuff" and my children. I share my dreams and my feelings and disappointments. I'm believing Him for the goals and dreams He lets me have. I'm believing that He will keep His promises even when I don't keep mine. When you want to know that you really believe you will tell others too. When we are afraid that God will make a fool out of us, we keep our "stuff" to ourselves.

I pray a powerful faith for you.

STUDY QUESTIONS:

1. What do you trust God with?

_____
_____
_____
_____

2. What are you believing God for?

___

3. Are you faithful? Explain. Do you submit to faith?

___

4. Do you worry? What about?

___

5. Do you speak with as if greatness is possible? Do you speak with belief?

___

As We Grow Together for Expectant Couples

6. Do you share the great things that happen?

_____
_____
_____
_____

7. Do you believe God will do what you ask? Do you ask believing that God will answer and provide? Do you ask believing that God will answer and provide?

_____
_____
_____
_____

8. Do you pray? Regularly? Do you have a prayer partner?

_____
_____
_____
_____

9. Do you fast? Regularly?

_____
_____
_____
_____

10. Do others know that you are faithful?

11. Do you think faith is important? Do you know that God expects you to have faith?

12. How do you measure faith? How does your measurement differ from God's?

13. Do your children know that you have faith? Explain.

14. Do you encourage others to have faith? Explain.

As We Grow Together for Expectant Couples

_____
_____

15. Do you know any scriptures about faith? Please list 5.

_____
_____
_____
_____

16. Do you move with faith?

_____
_____
_____
_____

Week Six — Monday

Faith: A Commitment to God

Hebrews 11:6

⁶And without faith it is impossible to please God because anyone who comes to him must believe that he exists and that he rewards those who earnestly seek him.

Hebrews 11:6

Read that scripture aloud. When I heard it in a sermon, after I heard it, there was silence in my own mind. It was as if God quieted everything around me so that I hear HIM say that – just to me.

Faith is a commitment to God. Faith commits us to God. Faith communicates to God that we believe, that we trust, that we hope, that we dream, that we have plans.

Faith is our plan to make God happy. My faith pleases God. It may be the only thing I have done correctly. The fact that I consider how to increase my faith pleases God. My faith validates His unrelenting commitment to me. My faith is a love relationship, where my faith shows I love Him and I am responding to His love. My faith communicates in a responsive manner that I hear Him and am ready for more of what He has for me.

My faith communicates that I test well and can receive larger blessings. I want God to know that I know that my faith, my belief, my trust, and my perseverance moves Him in amazing ways. My faith is tested just like everyone but the difference is that from my test, He has already foreseen the outcome. Sometimes I disappoint Him by faltering during a test but there's even a lesson in that. When I fail, He doesn't fail me. He tests me to stretch me and to grow me. Because growth requires change, I must be tested. The test is designed to increase my faith for bigger tests and so on.

He doesn't fail me, rather He continues to love me and keep me in His care.

My testimony includes my faith, expands my faith, increases my blessings and increases my opportunity to share.

Without faith, it is <u>impossible</u> to please God.

Faith is required. Faith is enough. Faith is an exhibit of hope. Faith is your expression of love. When I act and live faithfully, I demonstrate my love for God.

As We Grow Together for Expectant Couples

STUDY QUESTIONS:

1. Do you want to please God? Consistently?

   _____
   _____
   _____
   _____

2. Under what circumstances?

   _____
   _____
   _____
   _____

3. What do you want God to do in your life?

   _____
   _____
   _____
   _____

4. What do you want God to do in your child's life?

   _____
   _____
   _____
   _____

Week Six — Tuesday

Faith: Walk the Walk, Stop Talking

Matthew 14:28-31; Luke 8:43-48

[31]Immediately Jesus reached out his hand and caught him. "You of little faith," he said, "why did you doubt?"

[47]Then the woman, seeing that she could not go unnoticed, came trembling and fell at his feet. In the presence of all the people, she told why she had touched him and how she had been instantly healed. [48]Then he said to her, "Daughter, your faith has healed you. Go in peace."

Matthew 14:31; Luke 8:47-48

Get up and take action! Faith requires action. The story of the woman in Luke is the woman who had the issue of blood. She is very inspiring. She decides to make a move about her situation: she leaves home. She decides that nothing will stop her: she gets past the crowd. She determines her method of help: she grabs Jesus' robe. She accomplished her goal: she was healed. Great story, huh? It doesn't end there, though. Jesus NOTICED her. He felt her touch His robe because she had accessed His power. She didn't go unnoticed. He stopped what He was doing and asked, "Who touched me?" Initially, no one answered, then she finally confessed. Here is the blessing. Jesus speaks to her and encourages her to remain faithful and He offers her His peace.

When God grants you what you are believing Him to do, He is encouraging you to be faithful. Remember that God will be glorified when He delivers the promises He has made to you. When I am given the desires of my heart, I am immediately encouraged to remain about the items I am yet believing Him to deliver.

"Why did you doubt?" Such a powerful question, one we don't have a great answer for. We doubt because we forget and we fear. The implied statement that Jesus could've added, "Have I ever failed you? Why would I let you down, now? I am able to do all things." Jesus could've said anything proving that He was capable IF we believe. Jesus doesn't need to continuously remind us of what He is capable. However, we think He does because we keep demonstrating that we need reinforcement.

Faith requires action. Stop talking! Do what you need to do so that God can bless your work. God cannot bless anything that you haven't put any work toward.

Get up and take action!

AS WE GROW TOGETHER FOR EXPECTANT COUPLES

STUDY QUESTIONS:

1. What opportunities has God afforded you in order to demonstrate your faith to God but you failed profoundly?

   _____
   _____
   _____
   _____

2. Why did you doubt?

   _____
   _____
   _____
   _____

3. What action are you going to take to demonstrate your faith to God?

   _____
   _____
   _____
   _____

Week Six — Wednesday

Faith: Sometimes Alone

Genesis 12 - Genesis 22

[1]The Lord had said to Abraham, "Leave your country, your people and your father's household and go to the land I will show you.

Genesis 12:1

God told Abraham to leave his country, his family and GO! ALONE! Abraham was disobedient and took a cousin, Lot. At some point in the journey, they had to separate. Abraham had been distracted by the extra people he invited along. After all that was corrected, God could complete His work. Where is or has God leading you alone? Consider carefully your life and times in your life where God seemed to have you alone?

When we are alone, we can hear Him best. So when He has our attention, He is able to get us to work. Work is defined as prayer, fasting, forgiving, praising, and loving – all to Him.

God will fulfill His promises when you are faith-filled. I hear this among believers and "church-folk," but what does that mean for your life, your family and your children?

From the mother of two, take my word for it: You will never be ALONE again. ALONE starts with a re-prioritization of your own values, goals and time. ALONE leads to faith-filled. Faith-filled develops from spending time ALONE with God. As a mom, we spend our waking moments answering to the call, "MOMMY!" But God is screaming "Onedia," can I hear Him? Not all the time. When God wants to talk to you, can you hear Him?

From one mommy to another, ALONE happens when they, including your spouse, are asleep. Now Dads you may be wondering why am I addressing only mom and you should: the success of your family depends on her faith because of her time with God. Your prayer time and your study time needs to be established and announced and regular and respected.

During this time, God will meet you in your prayer time and in your study time so He can renew you and revive you and refresh you. Yes, I know you go to worship and Bible study and other church events and you are not alone. Your prayer life and study time is more critical now than ever. Fight for it. Prepare for it. Plan for it. With just as much detail as you have spent on preparing for the baby's arrival, create some private space for you and God.

Husband/Mate, you need prayer time and study time, too. Paint her space whatever color she requests.

STUDY QUESTIONS:

1. What does God want from you during that ALONE time? What does God want for you in that ALONE time?

_____
_____
_____
_____

2. When do you two pray together?

_____
_____
_____
_____

3. When will each of you study? When will you study together?

_____
_____
_____

4. How will you hold each other accountable to insure that this time is priority and protected?

_____
_____
_____
_____

Week Six — Thursday

Faith: Pass It On

2 Timothy 1:5-6; Romans 1:12

⁵I have been reminded of your sincere faith, which first lived in your grandmother Loris and your mother Eunice and, I am persuaded, now live in you also. ⁶For this reason I remind you to fan into flame the gift of God, which is in you through laying on of my hands. ¹²That is, that you and I may be mutually encouraged by each other's faith.

2 Timothy 1:5-6; Romans 1:12

You cannot share without experience. You cannot give what you don't have. You cannot pass on what you do not possess. I have discussed my education philosophy legacy throughout these pages but the most important is to leave my children a legacy of faith. I intend for Paul to be able to use me as an example. I want my children to experience faith because they see my faith in action.

Paul encourages Timothy "to fan into flame the Gift of God, which is in you." While faith is not in our DNA, this scripture begs the question: "Is faith hereditary?" Do we pass our faith on to our children? Did we get our faith from our parents? Certainly I can not prove that faith is hereditary or not, but what I do know is that faith is experienced and observed, rather than heard, taught, or discussed.

Faith is lived and experienced. Our children need to see us access the faith we possess in order to understand faith. My mother acted in faith but lived in silence. She never shared her concerns with me and rarely the outcomes of these concerns. I had to discern and decipher based on clues and conversations and silence. I really wanted to be there for her but couldn't because she didn't share.

Faith covers a multitude of areas of our lives – ALL. Not one of our issues is exempt from faith. God expects us to exercise our faith and act faithfully and respond in faith on all occasion. At all times. In all circumstances. In front of all persons – especially our children.

Faith is not foreign when felt on familiar fronts. Share your faith with your children.

STUDY QUESTIONS:

1. What does your faith teach your child?

2. With whom will you share your experiences?

3. How do you define faith?

4. Do you and God agree on that definition?

Week Six — Friday

Faith: An Action, Not Discussion

James 2:26; Matthew 17:20

[26] As the body without the spirit is dead, so faith without deeds is dead.

[20] He replied, "Because you have so little faith. I tell you the truth, if you have faith as small as a mustard seed, you can say to this mountain, 'Move from here to there' and it will move. Nothing will be impossible for you."

James 2:26; Matthew 17:20

Do you have enough faith? What is the size of your faith? A mustard seed is described as small. Jesus says that nothing will be impossible for us if our faith is at least this size – meaning that we don't need a lot of faith. At first glance, one may think that faith is sized or is measurable. However, when considering the possible metaphorical references, I am considering the fact that Jesus may have been explaining that faith doesn't have an actual size but rather an either you have it or not characteristic.

I also find that some people think they have faith but they really don't. They don't have it for many reasons: (1) they don't know what faith is, (2) they think about faith but there is no matching effort, and (3) they expect God to do all the work. The popular example is employment. The cliché is you don't expect God to knock on your door with a job if you never send a resume or send an application or make a call or even tell anyone you are looking for work.

A more applicable example is parenting. By faith, you have been given parental custody. However, you are on assignment. God has specific assignments for you as a parent. While I trust that she will grow to know God, it's my "work" to share God with her. It is my job to teach him to pray. It is my "work" to buy her a Bible, read it to them and provide a great spiritual environment for them. By faith, God will lead them to Him, keep them close and His will with them individually. God chose me to parent them by His will. When we realize that our daily work we do so that God can develop the results. While this may not seem as tangible as the defined job example, the parenting is more impacting and important. One doesn't simply change parents. Jobs change. Parents don't. Just a thought to consider: while you didn't pick one another as parent-child, you certainly don't want to be without one another.

This is most evident in adopted and foster children. They almost always want to know their real parents even though they have never had a relationship. The child just wants to know who was originally assigned to him.

Profound, huh? It doesn't matter who got the reassignment, they spend an unaccountable amount of time on the original parent.

Finally, why would God bless something you don't spend any time on? Faith requires work. Thinking, wishing and hoping don't count as work.

STUDY QUESTIONS:

1. What actions will be required to complete your God-given assignment?

_____
_____
_____
_____
_____
_____
_____
_____

Week Six — Saturday

Faith: The Final Word

Hebrews 12:2; Matthew 25:21

²Let us fix our eyes on Jesus, the author and perfector of our faith, who for the joy set before him endured the cross, scorning its shame, and sat down at the right hand of the throne of God. ²¹"His master replied 'Well done, good and faithful servant! You have been faithful with a few things. Come and share your master's happiness!'"

Hebrews 12:2; Matthew 25:21

Jesus is always our example for what we should do. Jesus is obedient and action-oriented and determined and energetic and discerning and forward-thinking. Jesus prays and is compassionate and caring and thoughtful and considerate and Jesus.

The goal for all Christians is for God to say, "well done, good and <u>faithful</u> servant! You have been faithful with a few things. Come and share Your Master's happiness!"

"Well done" are words the general human would love to hear from anyone, however God is the ultimate at this compliment. To hear His voice utter those words is the ultimate gift. "Good" means that I have been on good behavior. At least redeemable. "Faithful" is not a generally used term. The use of the words indicates a strong commitment through some unusual events and circumstances. Life constitutes that level of "faithful." "Servant" in the secular world is the lowest being. The Highest being in the spiritual world. When God uses servant and Onedia in the same sentence, He honors me for my service and obedience. In my service, I always have to remember that my service is to God rather than the person. He continues to admonish me to serve despite my personal feelings. To God, servanthood <u>and</u> the desire to serve defines leadership.

"You have been faithful" denotes long term faithfulness, not short-term, for-show "faith," a proven faith that exists when no one is looking, just what God sees.

"With a few things" indicates only what God defines as ultimately important. On His list are children, spouse, parents, and others He has called you to serve. God is not expecting us to do everything well (don't think this releases you from general accountability), but the ultimately important assignments is what the "few" defines. Does it mean your job? No. It does refer to the person or person(s) to whom you are assigned at work.

As We Grow Together for Expectant Couples

"Come" is an invitation with a promise of reward.

"and Share" is the completion of the reward for faithfulness.

"Your Master's happiness" is something at the top of the desire list and what we spend our time searching for and His happiness is the ultimate gift.

His gift of happiness is a certain reward for a mustard seed size faith over a few things.

STUDY QUESTIONS:

1. What do we need to learn from Jesus in order to please God?

_____
_____
_____
_____

2. What needs to happen for God to be pleased with my faith?

_____
_____
_____
_____

Week Seven

The Lessons Ahead

Your child also has the job of teaching you lessons. There are many lessons you have ahead. For those of you who may miss the lessons on the first round, there is great news. The lessons are presented until we get it. I promise. These lessons are for both of you. The lessons also expose your character traits and sharpens them. When this happens consider that education that is for you now, will later be used for them as well. God wastes nothing. God does not waste any opportunities for his glory to shine as well as for us to learn more ways to praise and glorify Him these lessons.

Lessons are multi-dimensional. These are the lessons we learn to move us forward. These are lessons we learn so we become closer to God. Then, these are lessons we learn so that we can reprioritize our lives. In all of these, the lessons are not new, but function as a reminder of how God really designed life.

Children do not possess fear. We teach fear based on our actions. Or lack of action. When we learn from their fearlessness, we learn to move forward and release our fears. Further, we learn to stop preventing them from moving forward. We also learn to stop teaching fear and start teaching abundant thinking and living. Finally, we are reunited with God's teaching of casting our fears on Him.

Next, there are the lessons which bring us closer to God and reestablishes accountability. As they grow older, they hold you accountable for your activities. We have a list of words that are off-limits. When my daughter hears us say one of them, she immediately says that she will tell our mothers, and that we know better. When the five year old in your life challenges your obedience to your rules, she reminds you that you are the parent and she is expecting your best. Her accountability also reminds you that you are accountable to God. Your parental relationship brings you closer to God.

Another lesson is remembering to dream, set big goals, and work hard.

Lastly, God wants us to leave our fears with Him. You must teach that to your child. In order to do that, you have to live that command.

You can only teach what you live.

AS WE GROW TOGETHER FOR EXPECTANT COUPLES

Sunday						Show her your prayer life early
						2 Chronicles 7:14; Luke 6:28; 1 Thessalonians 5:17; Matthew 5:44, 6:5

Monday						Document his many firsts
						Ecclesiastes 3:1-8

Tuesday						Hug her as often as possible
						Matthew 3:17

Wednesday					Make every moment count – each one is important
						Ecclesiastes 3:11-14

Thursday					Your marriage still requires the same attention
						Ephesians 5; 1 Peter 3:1-7

Friday						I rarely remember the disadvantages or hard times
						1 Corinthians 13:5; Matthew 18:21-22

Saturday					Your career and family sometimes conflict
						Genesis 1:26; 2:18; Proverbs 31:10-31

Week Seven — Sunday

Show her your prayer life early

2 Chronicles 7:14; Matthew 5:44, 6:5-13; Luke 6:28; 1 Thessalonians 5:17

[14]if my people, who are called by my name, will humble themselves and pray and seek my face and turn from their wicked ways, then will I hear from heaven and will forgive their sin and will heal their land.

[44]But I tell you: Love your enemies and pray for those who persecute you.

[28]bless those who curse you, pray for those who mistreat you

[17]pray continually

2 Chronicles 7:14; Matthew 5:44; Luke 6:28; 1 Thessalonians 5:17

Intuition doesn't come to an unprepared mind or heart or spirit. When she needs access to power and strength, she needs PRAYER, not mom or dad. Teaching her the power of prayer early gives her access. My daughter knows the power of access. She will pray anytime, for any reason because she has witnessed the power of prayer. When she says, "Let's pray." She stops and starts to pray. Children who learn to pray, never forget that access and power. They also know that they have unlimited access to God. This is when knowledge is the most powerful. They can pray without your knowledge, consent and interference.

The earlier you show her your prayer life, the longer you have to coach and check her knowledge. If you teach later, it will take longer for her to develop a prayer life and keep it consistent. As they grow up, they become influenced by outsiders and you need to set the foundation before the house is sitting there and you are trying to place the foundation under a built house. She needs to see prayer and hear prayer and pray before she has to rely on her own prayers or believe she is anyway.

As you show her that you pray, share with her the principles of prayer. Pray with humility. Pray sincerely. Pray consistently. Pray for those aspects for which you are thankful. Pray your adoration to God. Pray your confession to God. Pray your commitment to God. Pray for your friends. Pray for your family. Pray for your enemies. Pray for those who persecute you. Pray for your concerns. Pray for the desires of your heart.

Remind her that prayer pleases God. Show her how to pray out loud. Encourage her to pray with the family, her friends, and on programs at church. Pray at night with her. Pray for her in her presence. Listen when she prays for you.

STUDY QUESTIONS:

1. How can I humble myself in such a way that matches God's definition?

2. How hard is it to pray for those who persecute you?

3. What do you do so that you can pray for them?

4. How will you teach your child to pray for those who mistreat her and curse her?

Week Seven — Monday

Document his many firsts. Record all you can as many ways you can

Ecclesiastes 3:2

²A time to be born and a time to die.

Ecclesiastes 3:2

So when he's born, we do all the stuff for the birth and photos and baby book! We are excited parents! Then reality sets in and life gets back to hectic and then out of the "blue," someone asks you to see some pictures. The last picture is when he was six months old, now he is three years old. Then you are embarrassed because the picture is so outdated.

We take pictures on a quarterly schedule as a family: February, May, August and November. In February, my daughter takes the pictures for her birthday. In May, we take our generational photograph – my grandmother, my mother, my husband's mother, my daughter and myself. We also take a family photo. In August, sometimes optional, but fun pictures are taken. Finally, in October or November, we take holiday photos as well as my son's birthday pictures.

Pictures and memories are all we have to recall the many firsts and any stories that they generate. Also you'll want pictures to show them later and into their adulthood. I grew up taking pictures all of the time. My mother has volumes of my life on Kodak paper. I want the same for my children.

Firsts are non-repeatable and non-transferable. Do the most you can for all of your children equally. It does get harder when there's more than one but I encourage you to be diligent. I am always thinking about the future and I never want their lack of memories to be my fault. I also don't want there to be more memories of one child than there is of another.

To adult children, memories translate into love because of time spent as a family.

Consider your own situation. Recall your childhood – can you share it with your children? I can and my children will be able to as well.

AS WE GROW TOGETHER FOR EXPECTANT COUPLES

STUDY QUESTIONS:

1. How will you document her firsts?

_____
_____
_____
_____

2. How will you communicate to the other parent those firsts?

_____
_____
_____
_____

3. How can we operate to the level where we are in sync for the purpose of the firsts of the child?

_____
_____
_____
_____

Week Seven — Tuesday

Hug her as often as possible

Matthew 3:17

[17]And a voice from heaven said, "This is my Son, whom I love; with him I am well pleased."

Matthew 3:17

My daughter's favorite spot is in my lap. When I am sitting, she wants to be in my lap. Of course, this is great except I don't get to sit that often. Lesson to master: sit more often. That is easy to say if you don't have another child or a spouse or anything else. However, the reality is that we are all busy, but she should be third only to God and your spouse or self. We make two mistakes: (1) we put other "stuff" before our kids; and, (2) we put everything before ourselves.

First of all the airline's instructions are clear, yet ignored. Help yourself then help the child. Putting the air mask on her first could kill you, but placing yours on first will save you both. Secondly, when she <u>needs</u> you, you have to have enough fuel or emotional energy to help her. I have to hug her and comfort her and that requires energy that I have to save for her.

Next, we give our families the leftovers. I worked in customer service for years. When I get home, my children run from wherever they are and hug and kiss and yell my name. They are happy to see me and that I am home. They then expect to sit with me immediately – and sometimes I don't. They deserve my best. They thrive from my touch. I arrive home exhausted because I actually gave my best leftovers away at work. I only have mediocre leftovers to give them because I don't take time to care for myself.

I developed my new routine, which I'll share because I needed to be a great ME in order to be an awesome MOM! I take more baths with real bath bubbles and lotions and scrubs and oils. I take more time in the bathroom when I need to. I enforce my bathroom time boundaries with everyone. My hair, nails and feet have regular, standing appointments so that I look my best so I can feel my sharpest. I developed a wish list and mark off the things I receive, whether I purchase it myself or someone gives it me.

After all that, I sit down and <u>invite</u> her to sit in my lap. I invite her because it lets her know that Mommy loves her. It tells her that Mommy loves you and wants you to know it.

As We Grow Together for Expectant Couples

I need to hug her as often as I can because there will be a time when I can't. NOW is all that I have.

STUDY QUESTIONS:

1. How can you "sit" more often? Or whatever it is you need to do to spend more intentional time with your child?

___

2. How will you manage the "stuff" that will try to take your attention away from your child?

___

3. How will you remove the stuff that takes us away the time you need to spend time with your child?

___

4. How will they be first? How will you be at least move to third place in your life?

HIS WORKBOOK

_____
_____
_____
_____

As We Grow Together for Expectant Couples

Week Seven — Wednesday

Make every moment count – each one is important

Ecclesiastes 3:11-14

[12]I know that there is nothing better for men than to be happy and do good while they live.

Ecclesiastes 3:12

Time is precious. Time is unrecouperable. Time moves when you wished it would stop. Time is not rewindable. Yesterday is a distant memory. Tomorrow is not promised to you. The time you have is the moment you are in.

You have the same 24 hours as I do. What are you going to do with those hours?

I have some timing rules that you may find helpful:

(1) Washing machines, dryers, and dishwashers don't need supervision – turn them on at night or early morning.
(2) Saturday is not the cleaning day.
(3) Find a maid. If you don't think you can afford one, check you budget, eliminate something else and get a maid. The work 3-4 people do in 2-3 hours saves you time and you reserve your energy for those who need and love you the most – your children.
(4) Learn to go where they like for fun. It saves time for later.
(5) Establish time boundaries for bed. Their health depends on proper rest.
(6) Make a list before you leave home so that you don't waste time trying to remember where to go or what to buy.
(7) Schedule and respect your fun time. Fun and family don't just happen. It requires effort and energy and priority.
(8) Treat your time with care. Make your time special.
(9) Cook in bulk. Warm as necessary. Eat together. Cut off the television.
(10) Cut off the television. Yes, it was so important, it needed another mention.
(11) Read to your children as often as you get a chance.
(12) Spend your time wisely. Only spend your time on things that have a great return on your investment.

Capture your moments. You can't count them but you want and need every one of them.

In the movie, "Hitch," Alex says, "Life is not the number of breaths you take but the moments that take your breath away."

What takes your breath away?

STUDY QUESTIONS:

1. What are you going to do with those hours?

___

2. What takes your breath away?

___

3. Of these 12 rules, which four will be implementing first? Why? What rule is next?

___

Week Seven — Thursday

Your marriage still requires the same attention

1 Peter 3:1-7; Ephesians 5

⁷Husbands, in the same way be considerate as you live with your wives, and treat them with respect as the weaker partner and as heirs with you of the gracious gift of life, so that nothing will hinder your prayers.

1 Peter 3:7

Your marriage requires the same attention. Now more than ever you need to dedicate yourself to your marriage. Recall your courtship. Recreate those moments. Start interviewing babysitters so that you can keep your dates. Yes, you still need to date. You need time with your spouse – uninterrupted. You need this time to remember what your spouse likes and finds fun. Find time to converse about each other's thoughts and fears and needs and dreams. Remember how he likes his coffee. Remember her nail appointment. The little things mean the most.

Pray for each other and <u>with</u> each other. Keep your word – your promises. Women remember the promises men make and women fully expect those promises to be kept, without being reminded.

Men, don't forget what the scriptures say about your sacrificial love for you wife. SHE IS FIRST, after God. Husbands, your love equals her respect. When she respects you, she can love you. Without that love, you have no marriage – just a roommate and co-parent.

Ideally, you will "date" bi-monthly. These dates will be romantic and full of wonderful conversation, followed by wonderful lovemaking. If that's not your fantasy, that's great, however, whatever you desire for your date, make it happen. Your dates are an important quality time in your relationship. Take it seriously. Time goes quickly and if you have not committed any time to each other, you will be co-habitating with a stranger.

He still <u>needs</u> sex. She still <u>needs</u> conversation. Get creative. Be cooperative. Be flexible. Be committed. No whining. No excuses. Your marriage deserves time, attention and care. Your marriage is precious. Take care of it accordingly.

Make every conversation count. Ten minutes of uninterrupted daily face-to-face time with your spouse will kindle your relationship. Keeping all examples equal, treat your marriage like your vehicle. Rotate the tires every 5000 miles. Change the oil every 3000 miles. Wash it every weekend.

This is consistent and required maintenance, which you do so that the car is reliable and that the engine does not lock up. Each marriage is different but the basic principles are the same. Your marriage requires the same amount of attention.

STUDY QUESTIONS:

1. How will you spend time together?

___

2. Who is in charge of date night?

___

3. Who is in charge finding a sitter?

___

As We Grow Together for Expectant Couples

4. Are there some other boundaries which need to be understood to make this marriage have what it needs to be successful?

___

5. What is your definition of a successful relationship?

___

6. Do you and your spouse agree on that definition?

___

7. What does your mate need to be satisfied in the marriage/relationship?

___

8. What do you need to be satisfied in the marriage/relationship?

_____
_____
_____
_____

Week Seven — Friday

Your Grudge is Your Anchor

(I rarely remember the disadvantages or hard times)

Matthew 18:21-22; 1 Corinthians 13:5

[21]Then Peter came to Jesus and asked, "Lord, how many times shall I forgive my brother when he sins against me? Up to seven times? [22]Jesus answered, "I tell you, not seven times, but seventy-seven times.

[5]. . .(It) love keeps no record of wrongs."

Matthew 18:21-22; 1 Corinthians 13:5

Love keeps no record of wrongs. Tall order. Sometimes taller than others. But tall all the same. Yes, wives, it means put the scorecard in the trash. Yes, it is hard to do.

My friend said to me one day when you are having a hard time in your marriage: "Give your husband over to the Lord. It is not your job to fix him. He belongs to God. Give him back." Her statement took my breath away. I could barely breath. Give it up! Stop keeping a record of things gone wrong. You are still human. We all make mistakes. Forgive each other for EVERYTHING!! When you don't forgive, you stop the Lord from forgiving you. You also delay your own blessings.

In Ephesians 4:32, Paul also talks about love and forgiveness. It is hard to love freely, and openly, when you are holding a grudge. Holding a grudge is like a closed fist. When the fist is closed, you can't receive anything or give anything. Holding a grudge also stops your creativity.

Forgiveness is essential to growing as a person and in your marriage.

Love has to be able to flow freely in your marriage.

In the previous page, the scripture mentioned that certain actions would not "hinder your prayers," similar to this scripture, you forgive so that your prayers won't be hindered.

Keep forgiving! Yes, I know it is hard to do and it's hard to say. Keep forgiving! Forgiveness keeps the lines of communication open. Keep forgiving! Obedience to God means more than anything. God will honor your obedience. Keep forgiving! Your child benefits from this discipline. Keep forgiving! Forgiveness is key to a long and fulfilling relationship.

Just to clear the table of pre-existing issues, forgive yourself and spouse of <u>all</u> previous issues.

STUDY QUESTIONS:

1. Who are you holding a grudge against? Why? When do you plan to forgive him/her?

___

2. Practice saying the words **I forgive** out loud. How did you feel after saying it 10 times?

___

3. Forgive your mate. Family. Friends. Siblings. Explain.

___

4. Ask your mate how you can fill their love tank daily. How can they fill yours?

5. Ask it differently everyday. Share your results.

6. How will you help your child to forgive?

7. Who helps you to forgive?

Week Seven — Saturday

Your career and family sometimes conflict.

You may challenge your decision to return to work

Genesis 1:26, 2:18; Proverbs 31:10-31

[26]Then God said, "Let us make man in our image, in our likeness, and let them rule over the fish of the sea and the birds of the air, over the livestock, over all the earth, and over all the creatures that move along the ground." [18]The Lord God said, "It is not good for man to be alone. I will make a helper suitable for him."

Genesis 1:26, 2:18

God gave Adam a job. Husbands, you have a job. God provides for your family through you. In this century, half of last and the future centuries, women have become more independent and prominent in the workplace. God gave Eve a job, too. She was designed to help Adam. Wives are designed to help husbands. However, wives' jobs have changed since that time. Wives have evolved. Even though that is the case, husbands, your job hasn't changed. You need to have a plan for her to help you with. Yes, she can help you develop some of those plans, but the plans' foundation should be Biblical and established and shared with her.

I am that independent working woman who regretted not being able to stop working after my regular maternity leave. I was working when she took her first steps. I DECIDED that for the second child that I would work from home. I did that for eighteen months before I went back to work. There was definitely internal conflict with my strong desire not to return to work and the need for the money. Your current household budget may not allow you to stop working but it is necessary everyone to commit to the decisions made.

Several issues need to be considered: (1) if you can't currently afford to stay at home, what would it take? What would need to be cut so that you can? (2) What can each of you sacrifice to make it happen? (3) What work can you do from home? What independent businesses which target moms can you do so that you can stay at home? (4) What sacrifices can you make in order to stay at home?

If the decision to stay at home is important, then the sacrifice is inevitable.

Do whatever it takes.

STUDY QUESTIONS:

1. If you can't currently afford to stay at home, what would it take? What would need to be cut so that you can?

   _____
   _____
   _____
   _____

2. What can each of you sacrifice to make it happen?

   _____
   _____
   _____

3. What work can you do from home? What independent businesses which target moms can you do so that you can stay at home?

   _____
   _____
   _____

4. What sacrifices can you make in order to stay at home?

   _____
   _____
   _____

Week Eight

Life is Short – Do What Matters

Life is too short for worry, anxiety, anger, bitterness and grudges. I was pregnant on September 11, 2001. I was at home, going to work later but not really feeling great. I watched the tragedy happen. 2002 brought the one year anniversary of the day our national security was breached. I watched the special hosted by Diane Sawyer about the 65 children born of the September 11 tragedy.

Each day 63 women are reminded of the day which changed their entire lives. Best scenario: They were all at peace. They were perfectly happy. Worst scenario: They were unhappy. They had just had a fight. The fact is they were never able to make it right. Don't fall victim to that – make it right always.

When you consider your marriage and any issues, contemplate whether they are serious enough to hold on to. Ask yourself will it matter in twenty minutes. When you consider life's overall impact on you life, then some of the issues that really bother you may not be that important.

Life is too short. Do what matters. Decide what's important. Family time is ultimately important. What time is allocated to family? Are your dinners family style where everyone is at the same table and there is no television? This is true family time. How do you spend your weekends? Are your weekends dedicated to growing closer as a family? Do you take time to listen to the children? Can you modify your hours at work so that the family can eat dinner together?

There were several thousand stories from the survivors of 9/11. There is one that touches my heart the most. The owner of a company who was on floor 104 one away from the top, was walking his child to school the morning of the tragedy. His child asked him to walk her to school that morning. He agreed reluctantly because he would be late to work. He agreed and walked the child. He arrived at the area after the explosions. If he had been on time, if he had not walked the child to school, he would not be alive. It doesn't matter who he was, what he owned, the gender of the child, however, it does matter that he did what was important. We have 18 short years before they are no longer children. We need to make the most of each of those days.

What are you going to do to make the moments count and matter?

As We Grow Together for Expectant Couples

Sunday	Prayer is Power Romans 8:26
Monday	Love John 3:16
Tuesday	Timing Is Everything (Quality Time) Ecclesiastes 3:7-8a
Wednesday	Listening is a Skill James 1:19
Thursday	Quiet Time Psalm 1:2; 19:14; 145:5
Friday	Conflict Resolution is Essential Ephesians 4:26-27; Proverbs 15:1, 18; 17:9, 14
Saturday	Family Philosophy Joshua 22:5

Week Eight — Sunday

Prayer is Power

Romans 8:26

^{26}In the same way, the Spirit helps us in our weakness. We do not know what we ought to pray for, but the Spirit himself intercedes for us with groans that words cannot express.

Romans 8:26

Prayer is powerful. Beyond measure, prayer is extremely powerful. Prayer is our access to God. Unlimited access by praying to God in the name of Jesus is a provision made by Jesus' birth.

God is waiting on us to pray. He expects us to pray. He provides an avenue for us to pray. He has provided an intercessor, Jesus, who goes before us to pray. He also gives us the Holy Spirit to intercede when we don't know what to pray for. He is waiting for us to pray. He is concerned when we don't.

Prayer offers us several opportunities. We can adore God in our prayers. When we adore God, we simply love Him and the many ways that we love Him. Also when we pray, we confess our sins, reconciling our hearts to God. Sin separates us from Christ, so we need to be conscious of our sins and remember to confess them. God already knows what happened so go ahead and confess what will cleanse you of your sins and revive your relationship with God. Also, in prayer we offer thanksgiving; thanking Him for what He has done, but most importantly who He is. Then we pray with supplication. Align yourself with God, offering your best.

God is complimented by prayer and praise and scripture. When we pray, we tell God our needs, our wants and the desires of our hearts. The word says that if we delight in the Lord, then He will give us the desires of our hearts.

Prayer is powerful. Prayer is awesome. Prayer is required. Prayer does not have to be poetic, but sincere. Prayer is not perfunctory, but an honor we give back to God because of what He grants to us. Prayer is a form of praise. Prayer is also a time when God can talk to you. Prayer is when we can hear from God. We need to hear from Him.

Prayer is critical. Prayer is our lifeline to God.

STUDY QUESTIONS:

1. When do you pray?

   _____
   _____
   _____
   _____

2. What do you pray for? Do you share your prayer list with your mate? Explain why or why not.

   _____
   _____
   _____
   _____

3. Where do you pray?

   _____
   _____
   _____
   _____

4. How do you pray? What would make your prayer life better?

   _____
   _____
   _____
   _____

5. With whom do you pray?

___
___
___
___

As We Grow Together for Expectant Couples

Week Eight — Monday

Love

John 3:16

¹⁶For God so loved the world that He gave His only begotten son that whosoever believes in Him should not perish but have everlasting life.

John 3:16

John speaks of the most profound love one will ever experience. Jesus died for my sins and I wasn't there when He was flesh. As humans, we don't consider dying for those we do not know. We have reservations for those we do know <u>and</u> love. But without knowing me or you like He knew the disciples, He died for me. That's real love.

Will you die for them? Will you donate your organs to them? Do you <u>love</u> them? If so, how much? What are you willing to sacrifice? Is your love Conditional? Provisional? Earned? Real? Dr. Gary Chapman authored several books on <u>The</u> <u>Five</u> <u>Love</u> <u>Languages</u>. In these books, he defines love languages and shows that there are 5 and how to keep your spouse and children's love tank full. He also defines love tank. Love tanks and languages are subjective. Jesus is love is objective and unconditional.

Life is too short not to love fully and completely. We have a finite number of years here with our loved ones – make each one count. Love is required to have family as God designed. I may be selfish but I want to know that I am loved. My love language is time and conversation. When a person doesn't spend time with me, then I am not feeling the love they say they have for me. If we are not talking, I'm not feeling the love. For me, this is like air. To others, it's not important at all.

Children require time and equate time to love. There is an email where a boy wanted to spend time with his father. The father replied that he was busy. The boy left the room for about 20 minutes and then returned. When he returned, he asked his dad how much money did he make an hour. His dad replied, $20. He said okay and left the room and came back to the room with $20. He presented the $20 bill to his dad and said can I have an hour of your time.

If I could add an addendum to 1 Corinthians 13 as verse 14: Love is not busy and is not put off easily. When I want to say wait or mommy's busy, I am suddenly reminded of that email. I stop and address my children and give my love through my undivided attention.

STUDY QUESTIONS:

1. Will you die for them?

___

2. Will you donate your organs to them?

___

3. Do you love them? How much?

___

4. What are you willing to sacrifice?

___

5. Is your love conditional? Provisional? Earned? Real?

___

6. What is stopping you from loving completely and fully? Unselfishly?

___

7. Do people have to deserve your love for you to give it to them?

___

8. How do you like to be loved?

___

9. How do you know that the other person loves you?

His Workbook

_____
_____
_____
_____

Week Eight — Tuesday

Timing is Everything

Ecclesiastes 3:7b-8a

[7b]a time to be silent and a time to speak, [8a]a time to love and a time to hate.

Ecclesiastes 3:7b-8a

One of the many lessons that you will teach as a parent is one of the hardest – timing. My mother's lesson is "think before you speak." Although she said it dozens of times each week, I never fully understood until I started working. Timing in speaking is critical. Teaching that lesson requires honesty and fortitude and diplomacy. As I start teaching that lesson, I find that I have used the rule personally myself. My children repeat what they hear me say. If I want a parental report card, I listen to my children – grammar, vocabulary, tone, slang and attitude.

As I start sharing with my daughter how to think before she speaks, I have to remember that she is still small, five to be exact. At five, she has learned honesty but doesn't understand that honesty doesn't have to be shared with all parties. Caution is needed here because I don't want to inadvertently teach her to lie. I use "when we are honest we also are careful to be kind." This statement communicates that honesty is important and preserving the relationship, respect, dignity and integrity of both parties is equally important. Thinking before you speak and deciding to be silent requires wisdom and maturity. Teaching that lesson to a child also requires fortitude. You will have to say that same phrase several times in differing variations in order to make your point.

Teaching this lesson requires personal diplomacy and the ability to teach tact and diplomacy. How you say what you say is more important than the actual message. Tone and body language communicate loudly what you are saying and sometimes drowns your message.

Finally, love has its place and time. Love has interesting parameters. Timing and love normally don't work in the same platform. Although you can't time when you love someone, you can certainly work on your time to love those who deserve and desire your love. There is also a time to spend on love. Spend time with the idea of love.

Timing is everything. When you do something is as important as how and what you do. Using time wisely is equally as important.

STUDY QUESTIONS:

1. How will you teach the best use of time? How do you teach the value of time?

___

2. What is your parental lesson?

___

3. How will you teach lessons on respect, dignity and integrity?

___

4. What time do you spend on love?

___

5. What of your time belongs to others? How is that allocation determined?

_____
_____
_____
_____

Week Eight — Wednesday

Listening is a Skill

James 1:19

¹⁹My dear brothers, take note of this: Everyone should be quick to listen, slow to speak and slow to become angry,

James 1:19

Listening is a skill. Listening is a requirement in healthy relationships. Listening is required in all levels and stages and events in your life. Listening is the first step in love and conflict resolution. Listening is a very valuable skill.

Teaching my daughter requires that I speak slowly so that she can process what I am asking. Repeat what I need. Ask her if she understands what I need. Offer her the opportunity to ask questions. Sounds easy? It's a little more difficult than I explained.

The key to listening is connecting at some level of understanding. In order to effectively listen, I have to engage the speaker. When you are the parent, you have to engage the listener. I have to insure that she understands by using vocabulary she knows and using a tone she responds to well. Then I have to ask if she understood what I said. When she indicates that she did, then I know that we have communicated effectively.

The other component of listening is the follow-up and follow-through. The follow-up is me walking upstairs to be sure she is working on what was asked. The follow-through is her doing her share and knowing that I am holding her accountable for our conversations.

Now as the parent and even the spouse, you need to do some additional listening. I "listen" to my child's body language when she is talking to me. This body language communicates to me her happiness, fears, anxieties, joys, pains, excitement and her urgency.

As a parent, you also need to listen to their tone of voice. The tone will tell the second most important portion of the dialogue.

Lastly, I use my eyes and ears equally when I listen. I have trained myself to stop what I am doing to look at her when I listen to her. When I look at my children, I communicate that I am listening to them and I care about their concerns. When I do these things, I am also teaching them those same skills.

AS WE GROW TOGETHER FOR EXPECTANT COUPLES

STUDY QUESTIONS:

1. Are you an effective listener? Why?

_____
_____
_____
_____

2. Does your mate agree with you? Why?

_____
_____
_____
_____

3. Are you a patient listener?

_____
_____
_____
_____

4. Do you wait until the other person is completely done speaking before you speak?

_____
_____
_____
_____

5. Do you practice that listening is part of looking at the person?

_____
_____
_____
_____

Week Eight — Thursday

Quiet Time

Psalm 1:2; 19:14; 145:5

²But his delight is in the law of the Lord, and on his law he meditates day and night. ¹⁴May the words of my mouth and the meditation of my heart be pleasing in your sight, O Lord, my Rock and my Redeemer. ⁵They will speak of the glorious splendor of the majesty, and I will meditate on your wonderful works.

Psalm 1:2; 19:14; 145:5

By Gage's definition, meditate means to seek God in a quiet place with a receptive spirit, soul, heart, and mind. Further, meditation means taking time to reflect on what you have read, what you have seen, what you have heard and what God has for you.

Doing what matters should be priority. Quiet time needs to move to the top of the list. When do you sit down and let quiet cover you? When do you sit still without interruption? When do you seek the Lord and refuge in Him? When do you relax in the arms of the Lord?

When you become parents, your quiet time happens at a cost. Because you know that it is critical that you have quiet time, you will sacrifice other areas of your life so that you can have the quiet time you need. You <u>need</u> quiet time to refuel and reenergize yourself. You <u>need</u> that daily quiet time to reflect on the <u>great</u> things that God has done today. You <u>need</u> that <u>daily</u> quiet time so that you can resolve in your mind that today is passing and tomorrow is future. You <u>need</u> that <u>daily</u> quiet time to focus on God who redeems us from poor choices and bad consequences.

Don't feel guilty when you have your quiet time. You may self-inflict the guilt or maybe others will attempt to make you feel guilty. What is accomplished when you have your daily quiet time with God is worth far more than the guilt you will experience.

Quiet time with God is so valuable that it increases your effectiveness as a parent and a spouse. When you have had time to commune with God, you are able to maintain through life's ups and downs. You are closer to God because of this time. Remember the triangular relationship we discussed earlier, recall that we grow closer to Christ, we are growing for those we love. Further, your time with God becomes an example for those you love.

STUDY QUESTIONS:

1. When do you sit down and let quiet cover you? When do you sit still without interruption?

___

2. When do you seek the Lord and take refuge in Him? When do you relax in the arms of the Lord?

___

3. How do I communicate my quiet time to the family and friends so that everyone is on the same page?

___

4. How do you teach quiet time to your children? How did you learn?

___

AS WE GROW TOGETHER FOR EXPECTANT COUPLES

Week Eight — Friday

Conflict Resolution is Essential

Ephesians 4:26-27; Proverbs 15:1, 18, 17:9, 14

[26]"In your anger, do not sin. Do not let the sun go down while you are still angry, [27]and do not give the devil a foothold."

[1]A gentle answer turns away wrath, but a harsh word stirs up anger. [18]A hot-tempered man stirs up dissension, but a patient man calms a quarrel.

[9]He who covers over an offense promotes love, but whoever repeats the matter separates close friends. [14]Starting a quarrel is like breaching a dam; so drop the matter before a dispute breaks out.

Ephesians 4:26-27; Proverbs 15:1, 18, 17:9, 14

As you parent, there will come an occasion when you ask yourself what impression did I just make on my child? I learned this the hard way when one day my own words slapped me in the face. My daughter said something that was inappropriate at which point I promptly chastised her and then asked, "Who did you hear say that?" She responded, "You," quite innocently, I might add. I was appalled and embarrassed and completely enlightened. It was clear now that her memory was excellent. Her hearing was great too. And also that her sponge was absorbent. Our children are sponges, meaning that they catch everything in their presence. There is also an assumption they use daily: my parents are great examples and role models. As my parent, I should be able to repeat what they say and do. Is this a good assumption? Not always. As parents, we don't know it all, we make mistakes, and we are not perfect. Because of these facts, we need to be careful on how we approach these areas, such as anger, fear, and any other life pitfall.

Conflict resolution needs to be handled well at all times. Our children need us to show them on how to handle conflict. The same example could be used for you. What can you show your child? What can you shield from her? How do they see you resolve issues on the phone? At a restaurant? At home? With them? With their siblings? At the store?

When I shop with my children and the customer service is poor, I prepare to leave my potential purchase in order to avoid the situation. I now select where I take them and where I have stopped shopping in order to avoid having to be angry or upset.

Be careful as these situations arise. Remember that what you say cannot be reversed nor erased from her mind.

STUDY QUESTIONS:

1. What can you show her? What can you shield her from?

___

2. How do they see you resolve issues on the phone? At a restaurant? At home? With them? With their siblings? At the store?

___

3. How will you communicate and correct the mistakes you make?

___

AS WE GROW TOGETHER FOR EXPECTANT COUPLES

4. How will I show her how to settle and manage conflict? Without eliminating the relationship?

_____
_____
_____
_____

Week Eight — Saturday

Family Philosophy

Joshua 22:5

[22]"But be very careful to keep the commandment and the law that Moses the servant of the Lord gave you: to love the Lord your God, to walk in all his ways, to obey his commands, to hold fast to him and to serve him with all your heart and all your soul."

Joshua 22:5

What is your family philosophy? The family philosophy is based on your desired legacy, grounded by your beliefs and upheld by your daily activities. Your family philosophy has a long history as it has been passed on through all the generations in your family, then influenced by etiquette, social values, others, and Biblical principles.

How do you share your family philosophy? I share portions of it with my family as often as possible through conversation, discipline, behavior and faith.

I attended a wedding recently where I returned to my table from the buffet line. I noticed that the four seated people were not eating. Immediately, I prayed so that we could start eating. Before we picked up our forks, I asked the lady also at our table, "Are we using all of our manners today?" When I asked smiling, I already knew the answer. She replied, "Yes. They are almost done with the line. We can eat as soon as they are seated." My family philosophy included that etiquette. I chose to ignore it for a moment but I know the truth. Family philosophy provides instructions and guidelines for life and relations. A sample of our family philosophy is: "You have not because you asked not"; Family sticks together; Family spends holidays together; Family are concerned about each other; do not wear hats in the house or sunglasses; do not run with sharp objects; and, no singing at the dining table.

Some of these may be familiar to you, and if not, feel free to borrow them.

The point is to equip your child and family with an anchor and foundation for life which creates common ground.

Lastly, be prepared for the challenge when you steer away from the philosophy.

AS WE GROW TOGETHER FOR EXPECTANT COUPLES

STUDY QUESTIONS:

1. What is your family philosophy? How do you share your family philosophy?

   _____
   _____
   _____
   _____

2. How will you help those new in your home to understand your family rules and philosophy?

   _____
   _____
   _____
   _____

3. How will you support your mate when your family challenges her/him about the philosophy?

   _____
   _____
   _____
   _____

4. How will you support your mate when you do not understand why that is a rule/philosophy in the first place?

   _____
   _____
   _____

Week Nine

What Kind of Parent Would Jesus Be?

Jesus Christ was not a parent. Although unfortunate, He was not a parent but would have made a great parent. His character, attitude, and demeanor lends itself well to parenting. He is a also patient and kind and honest. Jesus would make a great parent. Using Him as an example, how can I be a great parent? I personally could use some tweaking of my parenting skills. Parenting gets complicated when issues are added such as financial, or marital or anything that keeps you from focusing on your parenting.

Child abuse is horrible but the actual child abuse takes place with majority women, Caucasian, ages 29-34, and middle class. The majority of the audience of this book fits the description of the average child abuser.

Why does that woman abuse her child? My best guess is based on my volunteer experience, she is overwhelmed with her life and all that her life entails. She doesn't have any help. Family doesn't live close. She and her husband haven't been on a date in months. She doesn't feel good about herself and she is too busy to know it. Take your life, add a child or two, add expenses to a budget that was already stretched, issues with employment, and stir, then you fit the description.

Parenting requires focus on the child. Jesus focused on us individually and collectively. When we are parenting, we have to prioritize what is most important between children and life. The children are the most important, if we forget or get distracted.

Jesus is a profound example of parenting. He knew how to discipline with love and compassion.

Parenting at the level God's prescribes requires love, forgiveness, intercessory, obedience, instruction, spiritual knowledge, and disciplinarian. Parenting also requires compassion, time, attention, research, resourcefulness. God demands your best investment in His children. We are the steward of His children. We need to consider what God has designed for that child and your family. That child carries on your great name. They may make your name great.

Parenting is the key to their success in life. How you treat them is how they expect to be treated in the world. As parents, we have full control of their self-image and self-esteem.

As We Grow Together for Expectant Couples

Sunday   Loving
                      John 15:9-14, 17

Monday   Forgiving
                      Luke 23:34

Tuesday   Intercessor
                      Matthew 6:9-13; 26-36

Wednesday   Obedient
                      Mark 14:35-36

Thursday   Teacher
                      John 7:16-17

Friday   Spiritual
                      Luke 2:46-47, 49

Saturday   Disciplinarian
                      Luke 8:24b

Week Nine — Sunday

Jesus Would be a Loving Parent

John 15:9-14, 17

⁹ "As the Father has loved Me, so have I loved you. Now remain in My love. ¹³Greater love has no one than this, that he lay down his life for his friends.

John 15:9, 13

Jesus had made the ultimate sacrifice. He died for all of our sins. He forgave those that ridiculed Him. He died for those who meant Him harm. He approached God on behalf of those who persecuted Him to have them forgiven. As a parent, Jesus would have transferred those same characteristics that He exhibited daily. Jesus loves without judgment. Jesus loves us in spite of ourselves, our sinful selves. Parents are judgmental and critical and overbearing and protective and possessive. Jesus demonstrates His love for us through His presence, deeds, teaching, wisdom, and service.

Jesus would chastise us gently. He would teach us so that we would not be chastised as often. He would influence our obedience. He would be easy to follow as a leader parent. Jesus seeks to understand rather than to be understood. Jesus used every miracle as a teachable moment. He would parent that way too.

Jesus would have the popular house, where all of the children came after school and on weekends. Jesus would sit around and talk to us about issues and scenarios we are experiencing. Jesus would be the parent who would volunteer at school and bring His child lunch on Fridays.

Jesus would love at a significantly different level because He is omnipotent, what regular parents need to help them along their parenting journey. Jesus loves deeply and would transfer that love to a child. Likewise, He would teach that same depth of love.

Jesus is the example of the greatest love because of the sacrifice He made to die for us.

Jesus is our ultimate parenting example for love.

AS WE GROW TOGETHER FOR EXPECTANT COUPLES

STUDY QUESTIONS:

1. How will we teach love to our children?

   _____
   _____
   _____
   _____

2. How will you love your child?

   _____
   _____
   _____
   _____

3. How will they know you love them?

   _____
   _____
   _____
   _____

4. How will you know that you love them?

   _____
   _____
   _____
   _____

5. What does your love look like?

_____
_____
_____
_____

AS WE GROW TOGETHER FOR EXPECTANT COUPLES

Week Nine — Monday

Jesus Would be a Forgiving Parent

Luke 23:34a; Matthew 18:21-22

[34a]Jesus said, "Father, forgive them for they know not what they are doing."

Luke 23:34a

Even on the cross at the brink of death, Jesus is asking for forgiveness to those who wronged Him. He intercedes on their behalf in an effort to save their sorry lives. And mine. Ours.

Jesus would be a forgiving parent. Jesus forgives and corrects with such mercy. As a parent, we benefit from His forgiveness. We also benefit from forgiving our children. Forgiveness frees you up from hate, lack of love, lack of engagement, and lack of trust.

The Bible says that we are to forgive seven times seventy. This is not a literal translation. This means to continue to forgive without limits. Jesus forgives like this. He made us in His image but we don't forgive in His image. We forgive based on pride, experience and benefit. We consider ourselves and those benefits first before we forgive to the benefits of others.

Forgiveness is not optional. Jesus forgives even those who persecute Him. We do not believe we should forgive if we believe we are justified. Wouldn't you agree that we do this? Because we do withhold our forgiveness, God can withhold His forgiveness from us.

What does forgiveness cost? It costs pride. I have to give up my pride when I forgive. This requires work for me. It costs God forgiving me, which is more valuable than my pride. It costs love. When two or more people are not more forgiving, then they cannot love one another. Love that is not reproducible is not needed. When love is at a sacrifice then time spent is affected.

Forgiveness is critical for personal growth and maturity. Lack of forgiveness stalls your growth and maturity. Forgiveness is essential to the relationship between people regardless of who those people are. As a parent, forgiveness is an essential to quality parenting.

STUDY QUESTIONS:

1. How will I forgive my child?

___

2. How will I teach forgiveness to my child?

___

3. How will I teach my child to forgive?

___

AS WE GROW TOGETHER FOR EXPECTANT COUPLES

Week Nine — Tuesday

Jesus is Our Intercessor as Parent

Matthew 6:9-13; 26:36

[36]Then Jesus went with His disciples to a place called Gethsemane, and he said to them, "Sit here while I go over there and pray."

Matthew 26:36

As I use my sanctified imagination, I would hope that when Jesus returned from His many recounted prayer sessions that the disciples inquired about the contents of Jesus' prayer.

As a child I was SUPER inquisitive so I know that I would ask Jesus, "Did You pray for me?" I would also expect an answer in the affirmative.

My mother prays for me, as I would expect her to. I have asked her for what do you pray. She prays for wisdom, knowledge, great decision making, favor, and financial stability. She prays for my sister and her children and grandchildren. She prays for my children and my marriage.

As a parent, you and your spouse should pray for your children daily. You are to INTERCEDE on their behalf. You are to seek forgiveness for their past. You are to pray for what they will face daily. You are to pray for their future. You are to pray for their day, that the paths they travel be safe and they are fruitful in their endeavors. You are to pray for their spouses and friends. You are to pray for their education and careers. You are to seek guidance for their future and their needs.

You are to pray for them daily before they rise. While they are sleeping, you are to seek God's face for your children. Jesus asked God for everything. Jesus shared with God EXACTLY what He needed.

You are an intercessor for your child. You need to remember your role. Just like Jesus intercedes on your behalf, you intercede on the behalf of your children. Your intercession penetrates the heart and mind and soul of their very being. Intercedes on their behalf.

STUDY QUESTIONS:

1. Do you pray for your child(ren)?

   _____
   _____
   _____
   _____

2. Do they know that you pray for them?

   _____
   _____
   _____
   _____

3. Do you pray for your mate?

   _____
   _____
   _____
   _____

Week Nine — Wednesday

Jesus Shows Us Obedience

Mark 14:35-36

[36] "Abba, Father," He said, "Everything is possible for You. Take this cup from Me. Yet not what I will, but what You will."

Mark 14:36

Jesus made the ultimate sacrifice. He died so that we may have life and have it more abundantly. When God told Jesus what He wanted Him to do, that Jesus would live for 33 years, sin-free but at the end of His earthly life He would die for my sins, Jesus said, "Yes, Sir."

Jesus watched God's plan and will for His life unfold. He walks us through each phase and each parable for use in our life. Jesus has God's bestowed powers but couldn't pass God's will.

Jesus is a lead by example leader. As a parent, I sometime lack this quality. Jesus asked to take this responsibility away. Then He totally submitted and surrendered to God. He told God that He will submit to God's will.

I need to do more of this. Jesus shows us obedient behavior modeling. He showed us how to be obedient and He shows us how to model obedient behavior.

God requires parents to be obedient as well. We are not exempt from obedience. Obedience shows God we love Him. When our children are obedient, they respect and love us. Parents often neglect the obedience because we are on a power trip. Parents are the ultimate authority in a child's life second to God. Sometimes we take the "authority" of our role too far. We extend and embellish our realm. We are not God to them. We have to obey God for their lives.

We are simply a steward of God's workmanship: "our children." As a steward, we are judged by God about how well we are handling our assignment. In order for that to work, we have to be obedient and use Jesus as our leader and example.

Negotiation is not applicable while obedient.

Study Questions:

1. How will we start to be obedient?

___

2. How will we teach obedience?

___

3. How will we discipline the lack of obedience?

___

As We Grow Together for Expectant Couples

Week Nine — Thursday

Jesus Is Our Teacher

John 7:16-17

[16]Jesus answered, "My teaching is not my own. It comes from Him who sent Me. [17]If anyone chooses to do God's will, He will find out whether My teaching come from God or whether I speak on my own."

John 7:16-17

I love math. I teach math. I tutor math. I advocate math. I love math because it is objective. Other subjects are subjective. I can prove a math problem to others who don't speak English and vice versa. God's word is the same way: His word can be proven and will be proven. When I teach, I am seen as the expert. I have been given credit for extensive knowledge in certain subject matters. I have been invited to speak in front of incredible audiences. These invitations have been great and the time is awesome. However, when I give false information then I sacrifice my "expert" designation.

Jesus suggests that we test His teachings through living according to God's word. When we live according to His word, then certain things happen. Jesus' teaching can be measured against a standard: God.

As a parent, we are expected to be an "expert" teacher. When we are wrong, we have to be honest. When we don't know, we need to say so. When we promise to find out information, then find it and relay that information.

As a parent, we are the first teacher. We are responsible for all the information that they intake whether they get it from us or not. We are responsible for their learning, education, and development. Jesus only authorized certain persons to teach. Jesus trained the teachers personally as disciples. His guidelines for teachers are clear.

Further, Paul states that teachers are accountable at a higher level. As a parent, we are responsible for their knowledge intake. We have to be selective about who pours into their lives at all levels. We are accountable for this. In addition, we are their ADVOCATE. We hold those educational contributors accountable as well.

Study Questions:

1. What do I need to teach this child?
   _____
   _____
   _____
   _____

2. How will I know what to teach and when to teach?
   _____
   _____
   _____
   _____

3. How do I insure that I am teaching correctly?
   _____
   _____
   _____
   _____

4. Who holds me accountable to teach what aligns with God?
   _____
   _____
   _____
   _____

AS WE GROW TOGETHER FOR EXPECTANT COUPLES

Week Nine — Friday

Jesus is Our Spiritual Leader

Luke 2:46-47, 49

[46]After three days they found Him in the temple courts, sitting among the teachers, listening to them and asking them questions. [49] "Why were you searching for Me?" He asked. "Didn't you know I had to be in My Father's House?"

Luke 2:46, 49

Effective parenting requires mutual accountability. Jesus sets the tone for spiritual leadership in our lives. Husbands, you are personally responsible for that spiritual leadership in our homes. Wives, you are to support his leadership. Husbands, your family is looking to you to set the agenda and follow-up on your plan. Husbands, do know that this role is heavily accountable and least appreciated but the most spiritually rewarded. Spiritual leadership requires a plan that influences growth, development and progress.

Husbands insure that regular prayer and Bible study and church attendance and ministry involvement occurs. He leads these activities by scheduling prayer and following through. He may not lead Bible study but he insures that his family attends Bible study regularly. He supports and encourages authentic ministry participation. He also participates in ministry opportunities.

The husband as the spiritual leader insures that his family is fed spiritually through all available means. Regular church attendance and fellowship with a local church is required for a healthy life. The wife enhances the relationship when the couple is spiritually aligned.

Jesus was about His Father's business at an early age. He committed to be the Jesus God called Him to be. Jesus provides an example for us to follow for spiritual guidance and leadership.

Study Questions:

1. What does a spiritual leader look like?

2. How do I insure that I am the spiritual leader of my home that God deserves?

3. What does God want me to teach? In what order?

4. How do I teach my child how to lead spiritually?

As We Grow Together for Expectant Couples

Week Nine — Saturday

Jesus As the Disciplinarian Parents

Luke 8:24b

[24b]He got up and rebuked the wind and the raging waters: the storm subsided, and all was calm.

Luke 8:24b

Jesus disciplines us because He loves us. I discipline my children because I love them. Whatever method you choose, your children respect you for discipline. Discipline is administered because of and with love. Discipline is also timely—not held as retaliation or used to reduce the child's esteem. Further, discipline corrects behavior and is not related to them personally or their feelings or future.

Jesus' discipline is complete POWER. He calmed the winds and raging waters with His voice. Even the winds obey Him—that's the power of His discipline.

Discipline requires consistency. Jesus models consistency. He disciplines us based on what we need for discipline. He does not discipline us the same. We are motivated by different entities. The consistency is key for the discipline to be effective.

These factors apply to our discipline: consistency, applicable, and timeliness. When I consider discipline, I ask myself is this an appropriate response for the "offense" or is this an attention stunt. I acknowledge that something inappropriate happened. I consider how many times this may have occurred before this offense. I decide whether the effects are lasting or fleeting. Lasting effects deem more severe discipline than fleeting effects.

Why did Jesus calm the storm? He taught several lessons: (1) Jesus possesses all power, (2) HIS POWER is far-reaching, (3) He reminded the disciples that faith in Jesus is required to be an effective disciple, and, (4) He uses anyone or any situation to demonstrate His point.

Consistent discipline delivers effective parenting.

Study Questions:

1. Am I a consistent disciplinarian?

2. Am I a fair disciplinarian?

3. Am I a conscientious disciplinarian?

4. Will my discipline teach the right lesson?

REFLECTIONS

REFLECTIONS

REFLECTIONS

REFLECTIONS

REFLECTIONS

APPENDIX

Your Testimony	213
The Names of God	215
Prayer Directions	216
Prayer Request List/Journal	217
Favorite Scriptures	223
Goals	230
Mission	232
Vision	235
Values	238
Dreams	240
Resources	243

As We Grow Together for Expectant Couples

YOUR TESTIMONY

Your testimony is your experience with God and the results of that experience. This includes your first encounter with Christ to your current life.

Consider the answers to the following questions to develop your testimony:

1. When did you first meet Christ?
2. How do you share how you met Christ with others?
3. What have your encounters with God been like?
4. What is your relationship with God like?
5. What danger has He kept you from?
6. What have you done that would have sabotaged God's work if He had not stopped you?
7. What has happened that you realized that only God was in charge to make this happen?

_____
_____
_____
_____
_____
_____
_____
_____
_____
_____

As We Grow Together for Expectant Couples

THE NAMES OF GOD

(1) Elohim: The plural form of *EL*, meaning "strong one." It is used of false gods, but when used of the true God, it is a plural of majesty and intimates the trinity. It is especially used of God's sovereignty, creative work, mighty work for Israel and in relation to His sovereignty (Isa. 54:5; Jer. 32:27; Gen. 1:1; Isa. 45:18; Deut. 5:23; 8:15; Ps. 68:7).

Compounds of *El*:

- *El Shaddai:* "God Almighty." The derivation is uncertain. Some think it stresses God's loving supply and comfort; others His power as the Almighty one standing on a mountain and who corrects and chastens (Gen. 17:1; 28:3; 35:11; Ex. 6:1; Ps. 91:1, 2).
- *El Elyon:* "The Most High God." Stresses God's strength, sovereignty, and supremacy (Gen. 14:19; Ps. 9:2; Dan. 7:18, 22, 25).
- *El Olam:* "The Everlasting God." Emphasizes God's unchangeableness and is connected with His inexhaustibleness (Gen. 16:13).

(2) Yahweh (YHWH): Comes from a verb which means "to exist, be." This, plus its usage, shows that this name stresses God as the independent and self-existent God of revelation and redemption (Gen. 4:3; Ex. 6:3 (cf. 3:14); 3:12).

Compounds of *Yahweh:* Strictly speaking, these compounds are designations or titles which reveal additional facts about God's character.

- *Yahweh Jireh (Yireh):* "The Lord will provide." Stresses God's provision for His people (Gen. 22:14).
- *Yahweh Nissi:* "The Lord is my Banner." Stresses that God is our rallying point and our means of victory; the one who fights for His people (Ex. 17:15).
- *Yahweh Shalom:* "The Lord is Peace." Points to the Lord as the means of our peace and rest (Jud. 6:24).
- *Yahweh Sabbaoth:* "The Lord of Hosts." A military figure portraying the Lord as the commander of the armies of heaven (1 Sam. 1:3; 17:45).
- *Yahweh Maccaddeshcem:* "The Lord your Sanctifier." Portrays the Lord as our means of sanctification or as the one who sets believers apart for His purposes (Ex. 31:13).
- *Yahweh Ro'i:* "The Lord my Shepherd." Portrays the Lord as the Shepherd who cares for His people as a shepherd cares for the sheep of his pasture (Ps. 23:1).
- *Yahweh Tsidkenu*: "The Lord our Righteousness." Portrays the Lord as the means of our righteousness (Jer. 23:6).
- *Yahweh Shammah*: "The Lord is there." Portrays the Lord's personal presence in the millennial kingdom (Ezek. 48:35).

- **Yahweh Elohim Israel:** "The Lord, the God of Israel." Identifies Yahweh as the God of Israel in contrast to the false gods of the nations (Jud. 5:3.; Isa. 17:6).

(3) **Adonai:** Like *Elohim*, this too is a plural of majesty. The singular form means "master, owner." Stresses man's relationship to God as his master, authority, and provider (Gen. 18:2; 40:1; 1 Sam. 1:15; Ex. 21:1-6; Josh. 5:14).

(4) **Theos:** Greek word translated "God." Primary name for God used in the New Testament. Its use teaches: (1) *He is the only true God* (Matt. 23:9; Rom. 3:30); (2) *He is unique* (1 Tim. 1:17; John 17:3; Rev. 15:4; 16:7); (3) *He is transcendent* (Acts 17:24; Heb. 3:4; Rev. 10:6); (4) *He is the Savior* (John 3:16; 1 Tim. 1:1; 2:3; 4:10). This name is used of Christ as God in John 1:1, 18; 20:28; 1 John 5:20; Tit. 2:13; Rom. 9:5; Heb. 1:8; 2 Pet. 1:1.

(5) **Kurios:** Greek word translated "Lord." Stresses authority and supremacy. While it can mean sir (John 4:11), owner (Luke 19:33), master (Col. 3:22), or even refer to idols (1 Cor. 8:5) or husbands (1 Pet. 3:6), it is used mostly as the equivalent of *Yahweh* of the Old Testament. It too is used of Jesus Christ meaning (1) Rabbi or Sir (Matt. 8:6); (2) God or Deity (John 20:28; Acts 2:36; Rom. 10:9; Phil. 2:11).

(6) **Despotes:** Greek word translated "Master." Carries the idea of ownership while *kurios* stressed supreme authority (Luke 2:29; Acts 4:24; Rev. 6:10; 2 Pet. 2:1; Jude 4).

(7) **Father:** A distinctive New Testament revelation is that through faith in Christ, God becomes our personal Father. Father is used of God in the Old Testament only 15 times while it is used of God 245 times in the New Testament. As a name of God, it stresses God's loving care, provision, discipline, and the way we are to address God in prayer (Matt. 7:11; Jam. 1:17; Heb. 12:5-11; John 15:16; 16:23; Eph. 2:18; 3:15; 1 Thess. 3:11).

Source: http://www.agapebiblestudy.com/documents/the%20many%20names%20of%20god.htm

PRAYER
A SHORT HOW TO GUIDE

The prayers which are most effective follow the following "rules:"

- It is a conversation with God.
- Be Honest with God.
- This is a relationship.
- God is to be praised, worshiped and glorified.
- God likes His word prayed back to Him.
- This is not a list of stuff you want.
- Think of more than yourself when you pray.
- Be authentic with God and yourself.
- Be prepared for people to ask you about your prayer life and faith.
- Do not worry about big words or long sentences.
- Please know that God is not taking revenge on others for you, and vice versa.
- Please prayer in the name of Jesus.
- There is no correct way to pray.

Scriptures on Prayer

Matthew 6:9-14

1 Thessalonians 5:17

Matthew 26:

John 17

AS WE GROW TOGETHER FOR EXPECTANT COUPLES

PRAYER REQUESTS
PRAYER JOURNAL

1. What are you asking God for?
2. What are you hoping God will do?
3. What are you expecting from God?
4. What has God already done to exceed your expectations?
5. What has God done to get your attention?
6. What has He shown about Himself and you?

_____
_____
_____
_____
_____
_____
_____
_____
_____
_____
_____

His Workbook

As We Grow Together for Expectant Couples

As We Grow Together for Expectant Couples

FAVORITE SCRIPTURES

Numbers 6:24-26

[24] The LORD bless you and keep you;

[25] the LORD make his face shine on you and be gracious to you;

[26] the LORD turn his face toward you and give you peace."

Jeremiah 1:5

[5] "Before I formed you in the womb I knew[a] you, before you were born I set you apart; I appointed you as a prophet to the nations."

Jeremiah 29:11

[11] For I know the plans I have for you," declares the LORD, "plans to prosper you and not to harm you, plans to give you hope and a future.

Psalm 8:1

[1] LORD, our Lord, how excellent is Your name in all the earth!

Psalm 19:14

[14] May these words of my mouth and this meditation of my heart be pleasing in your sight, LORD, my Rock and my Redeemer.

AS WE GROW TOGETHER FOR EXPECTANT COUPLES

Psalm 46:1, 10

^{1} God is our refuge and strength, an ever-present help in trouble. ^{10} "Be still, and know that I am God."

Psalm 119:11

^{11} I have hidden your word in my heart that I might not sin against you.

Psalm 139:14

^{14} I praise you because I am fearfully and wonderfully made; your works are wonderful, I know that full well.

Proverbs 3:5-6

^{5} Trust in the LORD with all your heart and lean not on your own understanding;
^{6} in all your ways acknowledge him, and he will make your paths straight.

Proverbs 23:7 (KJV)

^{7}For as he thinketh in his heart, so is he: Eat and drink, saith he to thee; but his heart is not with thee.

Habakkuk 2:2

^{2} Then the LORD replied: "Write down the revelation and make it plain on tablets so that a herald[a] may run with it.

Matthew 11:28, 30

^{28} "Come to me, all you who are weary and heavy-ladened, and I will give you rest.

^{30} For my yoke is easy and my burden is light."

Matthew 14:31

[31] Immediately Jesus reached out his hand and caught him. "You of little faith," he said, "why did you doubt?"

Matthew 22:37

[37] Jesus replied: "'Love the Lord your God with all your heart and with all your soul and with all your mind.

Matthew 28:19-20

[19] Therefore go and make disciples of all nations, baptizing them in[a] the name of the Father and of the Son and of the Holy Spirit, [20] and teaching them to obey everything I have commanded you. And surely I am with you always, to the very end of the age."

Luke 9:24

[23] Then he said to them all: "If anyone would come after me, he must deny himself and take up his cross daily and follow me. [24] For whoever wants to save his life will lose it, but whoever loses his life for me will save it.

Luke 23:34

[34] Jesus said, "Father, forgive them, for they do not know what they are doing."[a] And they divided up his clothes by casting lots.

John 1:1-2

[1] In the beginning was the Word, and the Word was with God, and the Word was God. [2] He was with God in the beginning.

As We Grow Together for Expectant Couples

John 3:16

[16] "For God so loved the world that he gave his one and only Son,[a] that whoever believes in him shall not perish but have eternal life.

John 3:30

[30] He must become greater; I must become less.

John 11:35

[35] Jesus wept.

Romans 8:26

[26] In the same way, the Spirit helps us in our weakness. We do not know what we ought to pray for, but the Spirit himself intercedes for us with groans that words cannot express.

1 Corinthians 10:13

[13] No temptation has seized you except what is common to man. And God is faithful; he will not let you be tempted beyond what you can bear. But when you are tempted, he will also provide a way out so that you can stand up under it.

Galatians 5:22-23

[22] But the fruit of the Spirit is love, joy, peace, patience, kindness, goodness, faithfulness, [23] gentleness and self-control. Against such things there is no law.

Ephesians 3:14-21

[14] For this reason I kneel before the Father, [15] from whom his whole family[a] in heaven and on earth derives its name. [16] I pray that out of his glorious riches he may strengthen you with power through his Spirit in your inner being, [17] so that Christ may dwell in your hearts through faith. And I pray that you, being rooted and established in love, [18] may have power, together with all the saints, to grasp how wide and long and high and deep is the love of Christ, [19] and to know this love that surpasses knowledge—that you may be filled to the measure of all the fullness of God. [20] Now unto him who is able to do immeasurably more than all we ask or imagine, according to his power that is at work within us, [21] to him be glory in the church and in Christ Jesus throughout all generations, for ever and ever! Amen.

Ephesians 4:26-27

[26] "In your anger do not sin"[a]: Do not let the sun go down while you are still angry, [27] and do not give the devil a foothold.

Ephesians 4:32

[32] Be kind and compassionate to one another, forgiving each other, just as in Christ God forgave you.

Philippians 4:7

[7] And the peace of God, which transcends all understanding, will guard your hearts and your minds in Christ Jesus.

Philippians 4:13-17

[13] I can do everything through him who gives me strength. [14] Yet it was good of you to share in my troubles. [15] Moreover, as you Philippians know, in the early days of your acquaintance with the gospel, when I set out from Macedonia, not one church shared with me in the matter of giving and receiving, except you only; [16] for even when I

was in Thessalonica, you sent me aid again and again when I was in need. [17] Not that I am looking for a gift, but I am looking for what may be credited to your account.

Colossians 3:23

[23] Whatever you do, work at it with all your heart, as working for the Lord, not for men,

1 Thessalonians 5:17

[17] pray continually;

Hebrews 11:6

[6] And without faith it is impossible to please God, because anyone who comes to him must believe that he exists and that he rewards those who earnestly seek him.

Hebrews 13:5b

[5] Keep your lives free from the love of money and be content with what you have, because God has said, "Never will I leave you; never will I forsake you."

James 1:2-5

[2] Consider it pure joy, my brothers, whenever you face trials of many kinds, [3] because you know that the testing of your faith develops perseverance. [4] Perseverance must finish its work so that you may be mature and complete, not lacking anything. [5] If any of you lacks wisdom, he should ask God, who gives generously to all without finding fault, and it will be given to him.

Jude 24

[24] Now unto him that is able to keep you from falling, and to present you faultless before the presence of his glory with exceeding joy,

Revelation 3:16

[16] So, because you are lukewarm—neither hot nor cold—I am about to spit you out of my mouth.

As We Grow Together for Expectant Couples

GOALS

goal [gohl] *noun*

the result or achievement toward <u>which</u> effort is directed; aim; end.

The questions that you answer when developing goals are as follows:

1. What do I want to accomplish for God, with God, because of God?
2. When do I want to accomplish this by? What does God's timing look like?
3. Who is going to help me and hold me accountable? Who has God sent my way for this matter?
4. What do you do when you do not meet the goals as planned? What will God do in the meantime?
5. Who do you share your successes with? How will God use my achievement to help others?

GOALS

Goals	By When	Who

MISSION STATEMENT

A personal mission statement is based on habit 2 of <u>7 Habits of Highly Effective People</u> called begin with the end in mind. In ones life, the most effective way to begin with the end in mind is to develop a mission statement one that focuses what you want to be in terms of character and what you want to do in reference to contribution of achievements. Writing a mission statement can be the most important activity an individual can take to truly lead ones life.

Victor Hugo once said there is nothing as powerful as an idea whose time has finally come, you may call it a credo, a philosophy, you may call it a purpose statement, it's not as important as to what you call it, no it's how you define your definition. That mission and vision statement is more powerful, more significant, more influential, than the baggage of the past, or even the accumulated noise of the present.

What is a mission statement you ask? Personal mission statements based on correct principles are like a personal constitution, the basis for making major, life-directing decisions, the basis for making daily decisions in the midst of the circumstances and emotions that affect our lives.

Your statement may be a few words or several pages, but it is not a "to do" list. It reflects your uniqueness and must speak to you powerfully about the person you are and the person you are becoming.

Why should you write a personal mission statement?

Numerous experts on leadership and personal development emphasize how vital it is for you to craft your own personal vision for your life. Warren Bennis, Stephen Covey, Peter Senge, and others point out that a powerful vision can help you succeed far beyond where you'd be without one. That vision can propel you and inspire those around you to reach their own dreams.

Q: How do I go about creating my Personal Mission Statement?

A: A Mission Statement is defined as having goals and a deadline. This is opposed to the notion that a Mission Statement is just a bunch of flowery, general phrases like, "I will be the best business person I can be."

What should you include when writing a great personal mission statement?

- describe your best characteristics and how you express them
- have specific, measurable outcomes (or goals)
- have a deadline — for example, December 31st 2012, or a year from today.

When Stephen Covey talks about 'mission statement' in this quote, he is referring to the articulation of your life purpose. "If you don't set your goals based upon your Mission Statement, you may be climbing the ladder of success only to realize, when you get to the top, you're on the WRONG BUILDING." **Stephen Covey – 7 Habits of Highly Effective People.**

Mission Statement Example – Poor (It's more like a Vision Statement)

"I aspire to start my own business. I want to help others and be a better businesswoman. I will deliver the best food with the highest service levels." Jane

Mission Statement Example – Better

"I will start my business within 3 months and plan to grow it to $500,000 in revenues within a year. Using this success, my staff and I will spread the word to local schools and businesses about eco-friendly food production in order that we reach at least 100 people within the same time frame. My purpose will be to massively add value to our local community in measurable ways that have a real impact on people's health now and in the future," Jane.

What to do with your Mission Statement?

So now we have a mission, we can set a range of goals on the road to achieving your outcomes and dreams. Your values are clarified and should be in line with the goals you want to achieve in life so you should find it easier to make decisions and to do the "right thing" because you can simply ask yourself, "Will this help me achieve my mission?"

You can even put your mission statement in an area where your family or even co-workers will see it. For, a mission statement defines who you are and what you stand for. This lets people see how you think and feel, which in turn, will help them respect, think and act in line with your values too.

MISSION STATEMENT

VISION STATEMENT

A personal vision/mission statement is the framework for creating a powerful life.

Your personal vision statement provides the direction necessary to guide the course of your days and the choices you make about your life.

The idea is to craft a broad based idea about your life and what will really make it exciting and fulfilling, that's your life vision.

From the vision, you craft a more focused and action orientated "mission" statement based on "purpose." And finally you get to a list of goals, wishes, desires and needs.

In his book 'The Success Principles,' Jack Canfield tells us that in order to create a balanced and successful life; your vision needs to include the following seven areas:

1. work and career
2. finances
3. recreation and free time
4. health and fitness
5. relationships
6. personal goals
7. contribution to the larger community

It does not include the distinctive ways that you intend to accomplish your purpose.

Why Write a Personal Vision Statement?

To express:
- your purpose
- your life's dream
- your core values & beliefs
- what you want for yourself
- what you want to contribute to others
- what you want to be

Characteristics of a Vision Statement:

- Engages your heart & spirit
- Taps into embedded concerns & needs
- Asserts what you want to create
- Is something worth going for
- Provides meaning to the work you do
- Is a little cloudy and grand
- Is simple
- Is a living document
- Provides a starting place from which to get more specificity
- Is based on quality and dedication

Key Elements of a Vision Statement:

- Written down and referred to daily
- Written in present tense, as if it has already been completed
- Includes a variety of activities and time frames
- Filled with descriptive details that anchor it to reality

What Visions Are Not:

- A mission statement: "Why do we exist now?"
- A strategic plan: "How do we plan to get there?"
- A set of objectives: "We will accomplish X by Y time to Z% target audience."

Use these questions to guide your thoughts:

- What are the ten things you most enjoy doing? Be honest. These are the ten things without which your weeks, months, and years would feel incomplete.
- What three things must you do every single day to feel fulfilled in your work?
- What are your five-six most important values?
- Your life has a number of important facets or dimensions, all of which deserve some attention in your personal vision statement.
- Write one important goal for each of them: physical, spiritual, work or career, family, social relationships, financial security, mental improvement and attention, and fun.
- If you never had to work another day in your life, how would you spend your time instead of working?
- When your life is ending, what will you regret not doing, seeing, or achieving?
- What strengths have other people commented on about you and your accomplishments? What strengths do you see in yourself?

VISION STATEMENT

VALUES STATEMENT

A personal **value** is <u>absolute or relative and ethical value</u>, the assumption of which can be the basis for ethical action. A *value system* is a set of consistent <u>values</u> and measures. A *principle value* is a foundation upon which other values and measures of <u>integrity</u> are based.

Some values are physiologically determined and are normally considered objective, such as a desire to avoid physical pain or to seek pleasure. Other values are considered <u>subjective</u>, vary across individuals and cultures, and are in many ways aligned with <u>belief</u> and belief systems. Types of values include <u>ethical</u>/<u>moral</u> values, <u>doctrinal</u>/<u>ideological</u> (religious, political) values, <u>social</u> values, and <u>aesthetic</u> values. It is debated whether some values that are not clearly physiologically determined, such as <u>altruism</u>, are <u>intrinsic</u>, and whether some, such as acquisitiveness, should be classified as <u>vices</u> or <u>virtues</u>. Values have been studied in various disciplines: <u>anthropology</u>, <u>behavioral economics</u>, <u>business ethics</u>, <u>corporate governance</u>, <u>moral philosophy</u>, <u>political sciences</u>, <u>social psychology</u>, <u>sociology</u> and <u>theology</u> to name a few.

Values can be defined as broad preference concerning appropriate courses of action or outcomes. As such, values reflect a person's sense of right and wrong or what "ought" to be. "Equal rights for all", "Excellence deserves admiration", and "People should be treated with respect and dignity" are representative of values. Values tend to influence attitudes and behavior.

VALUES STATEMENT

AS WE GROW TOGETHER FOR EXPECTANT COUPLES

DREAMS LIST

As We Grow Together for Expectant Couples

RESOURCES

www.onediagage.com

As We Grow Together Daily Devotional for Expectant Couples

As We Grow Together Prayer Journal for Expectant Couples

The Blue Print: Poetry for the Soul

From Two to One: The Notebook for Couples

In Purple Ink: Poetry for the Spirit

Living a Whole Life: Sermons which Prompt, Provoke and Promote Life

Love Letters to God from a Teenage Girl

The Measure of a Woman: The Details of Her Soul

The Notebook: For Me, About Me, By Me

The Notebook for the Christian Teen

On This Journey Daily Devotional for Young People

On This Journey Prayer Journal for Young People

One Day More Than We Deserve Daily Devotional for the Growing Christian

One Day More Than We Deserve Prayer Journal for the Growing Christian

Promises, Promises: A Christian Novel

Tools for These Times: Timely Sermons for Uncertain Times

With An Anointed Voice: The Power of Prayer

Yielded and Submitted: A Woman's Journey for a Life Dedicated to God

Yielded and Submitted: A Woman's Journey for a Life Dedicated to God Prayers and Journal

Yielded and Submitted: A Woman's Journey for a Life Dedicated to God An Intimate Study

The Power of a Praying Woman Stormie Omartian

The Power of a Praying Wife Stormie Omartian

Discerning the Voice of God Priscilla Shrirer

Kingdom Woman Tony Evans and Crystal Evans Hurst

As We Grow Together for Expectant Couples

ACKNOWLEDGEMENTS

God, thank You for Your plans for me. Thank You for *As We Grow Together: The Workbook for Expectant Couples,* and choosing me to complete Your project. I just want to please You, God. Thank You for continuing to anoint me and to invest in me and my gifts, which keep surprising me. Thank You for loving and forgiving me.

Hillary and Nehemiah, thank you for supporting me and my endeavors. Thank you for loving me, especially when I do nothing without a pen and a clipboard, thank you for enduring my late nights, your ideas, the sounding board, the love and the support. Thank you for celebrating our legacy.

To Sanya Skillern. Thank you for your accountability. Thank you for reading and answering the questions and editing those errors and clarifying those unclear areas. Your time, effort and contribution mean a lot to me.

To my prayer partners and to my accountability partners, thank you for the long talks and the powerful prayers and the encouragement.

To the readers who this will reach and empower and touch and affect, may these words empower you and help you reach some resolve. May you be inspired to achieve your goals and dreams. May you enhance your relationship with God so that your other relationships will also improve. May you enhance your self-esteem through prayer and study. May you have courage and peace. Share love the best you can until you can share love without reservation.

AS WE GROW TOGETHER FOR EXPECTANT COUPLES

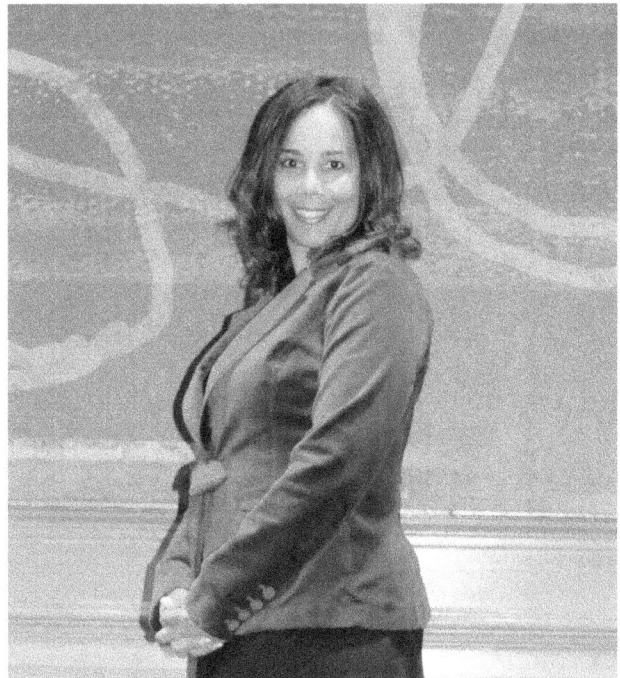

ABOUT THE MOM

The author believes that questions help you to grow and create the appropriate amount of challenge.

Do not hesitate to ask, to engage at a high level of participation, anticipating God's best for you!

@onediangage (twitter) ♦ onediagage@onediagage.com ♦ facebook.com/onediagageministries

youtube.com/onediagage ♦ blogtalkradio.com/onediagage ♦ ongage (instagram)

www.onediagage.com

As We Grow Together for Expectant Couples

HIS WORKBOOK

PREACHER ♦ TEACHER ♦ FACILITATOR

CONFERENCE SPEAKER ♦ PANELIST ♦ WORKSHOP LEADER

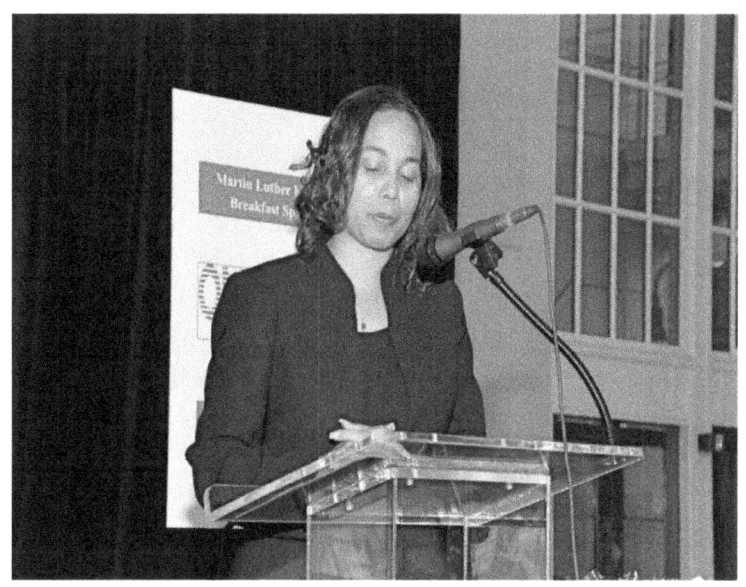

To invite Ms. Gage to speak at your church, couples ministry, youth group, or youth ministry,

Please contact us at: www.onedigage.com

@onediangage (twitter) ♦ onediagage@onediagage.com ♦ facebook.com/onediagageministries

youtube.com/onediagage ♦ blogtalkradio.com/onediagage

As We Grow Together for Expectant Couples

Publishing

Do you have a book you want to write, but do not know what to do?

Do you have a book you need to publish but do not know how to start?

Would publishing move your career forward?

Let us help

onediagage@purpleink.net ♦ www.purpleink.net

713.705.5530 ♦ 512.715.4243

www.ingramcontent.com/pod-product-compliance
Lightning Source LLC
Chambersburg PA
CBHW081346080526
44588CB00016B/2391